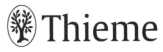

# Vasculature of the Brain and Cranial Base

Variations in Clinical Anatomy

2nd Edition

**Walter Grand, MD**
Clinical Professor of Neurosurgery and Anatomical Sciences
Department of Neurosurgery
School of Medicine and Biomedical Sciences
University at Buffalo
Buffalo, New York

**L. Nelson Hopkins III, MD**
Distinguished Professor and Chairman, Neurosurgery and Radiology
University at Buffalo
Founder, Gates Vascular Institute and Jacobs Institute
Buffalo, New York

**Adnan H. Siddiqui, MD**
Vice-Chairman and Professor
Director of Neuroendovascular Fellowship
Director of Research
Department of Neurosurgery
University at Buffalo
Director of Neurosurgical Stroke Service, Kaleida Health
Director, Training and Education, Jacobs Institute
Buffalo, New York

**J Mocco, MD, MS**
Professor and Vice-Chair for Education
Director, The Cerebrovascular Center
Department of Neurological Surgery
Mount Sinai Health System
New York, New York

352 illustrations

Thieme
New York • Stuttgart • Delhi • Rio de Janeiro

Executive Editor: Timothy Hiscock
Managing Editor: Elizabeth Palumbo
Director, Editorial Services: Mary Jo Casey
Production Editor: Kenneth L. Chumbley
International Production Director: Andreas Schabert
Senior Vice President, Editorial and E-Product Development:
    Vera Spillner
International Marketing Director: Fiona Henderson
International Sales Director: Louisa Turrell
Director of Sales, North America: Mike Roseman
Senior Vice President and Chief Operating Officer: Sarah Vanderbilt
President: Brian D. Scanlan

Illustrations by Paul H. Dressel
Art Design and Photography by Paul H. Dressel and Walter Grand, MD

**Library of Congress Cataloging-in-Publication Data**
Grand, Walter, author.
Vasculature of the brain and cranial base : variations in clinical
anatomy / Walter Grand, L. Nelson Hopkins, Adnan Siddiqui,
J Mocco. — 2nd edition.
    p. ; cm.
Includes bibliographical references and index.
ISBN 978-1-60406-885-6 (alk. paper) — ISBN 978-1-60406-886-3
(eBook)
I. Hopkins, L. N., author. II. Siddiqui, Adnan (Professor of neurosurgery and radiology), author. III. Mocco, J., author. IV. Title.
[DNLM: 1. Brain—blood supply—Atlases. 2. Cerebrovascular Circulation—Atlases. 3. Skull—blood supply—Atlases. WL 17]
QP376
612.8'240222—dc23                                    2015018650

© 2016 Thieme Medical Publishers, Inc.
Thieme Publishers New York
333 Seventh Avenue, New York, NY 10001 USA
+1 800 782 3488, customerservice@thieme.com

Thieme Publishers Stuttgart
Rüdigerstrasse 14, 70469 Stuttgart, Germany
+49 [0]711 8931 421, customerservice@thieme.de

Thieme Publishers Delhi
A-12, Second Floor, Sector-2, Noida-201301
Uttar Pradesh, India
+91 120 45 566 00, customerservice@thieme.in

Thieme Publishers Rio de Janeiro, Thieme Publicações Ltda.
Edifício Rodolpho de Paoli, 25º andar
Av. Nilo Peçanha, 50 – Sala 2508
Rio de Janeiro 20020-906, Brasil
+55 21 3172 2297

Cover design: Thieme Publishing Group
Typesetting by Prairie Papers, USA

Printed in India by Replika Press Pvt. Ltd.           5 4 3 2 1

ISBN 978-1-60406-885-6

Also available as an e-book:
eISBN 978-1-60406-886-3

**Important note:** Medicine is an ever-changing science undergoing continual development. Research and clinical experience are continually expanding our knowledge, in particular our knowledge of proper treatment and drug therapy. Insofar as this book mentions any dosage or application, readers may rest assured that the authors, editors, and publishers have made every effort to ensure that such references are in accordance with **the state of knowledge at the time of production of the book.**

Nevertheless, this does not involve, imply, or express any guarantee or responsibility on the part of the publishers in respect to any dosage instructions and forms of applications stated in the book. **Every user is requested to examine carefully** the manufacturers' leaflets accompanying each drug and to check, if necessary in consultation with a physician or specialist, whether the dosage schedules mentioned therein or the contraindications stated by the manufacturers differ from the statements made in the present book. Such examination is particularly important with drugs that are either rarely used or have been newly released on the market. Every dosage schedule or every form of application used is entirely at the user's own risk and responsibility. The authors and publishers request every user to report to the publishers any discrepancies or inaccuracies noticed. If errors in this work are found after publication, errata will be posted at www.thieme.com on the product description page.

Some of the product names, patents, and registered designs referred to in this book are in fact registered trademarks or proprietary names even though specific reference to this fact is not always made in the text. Therefore, the appearance of a name without designation as proprietary is not to be construed as a representation by the publisher that it is in the public domain.

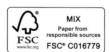

# Contents

# Preface

The 2nd edition, as was the 1st, is based on hundreds of dissections of the brain and cranial base. It is the culmination of 40 years of my personal study of neurovascular anatomy and relies primarily on morbid anatomy. Frequently, even the most experienced neurosurgeon, cannot be sure of the precise anatomy, nor can the neuroradiologist be sure of the intricacies of the vasculature on an angiographic film. This is precisely the point! The illustrations and figures are meant to expand the "vision" of the neurosurgeon in the surgical field and sharpen the perception of the neuroradiologist, neuroendovascular interventionlist, and neurologist.

Nothing is more striking in neurovascular anatomy than the myriad varieties of branching and configuration of vessels. Even after compiling numerous variations on a vessel in the brain, one can still say that two vessels never look exactly alike. The more closely one looks at the subtleties of the vasculature of the brain, the more differences one sees. I have tried to consolidate the classifications of variations of the vasculature of the brain and cranial base and, in some cases, unavoidably had to simplify variations for clarity. The neuroendovascular correlates at the end of each chapter add a dynamic and invaluable addition to this 2nd edition text.

*Walter Grand, MD*
*Senior Author*

# Introduction

This 2nd edition includes a neuroendovascular correlative section at the end of each anatomical chapter, which adds a nice clinical dimension to the anatomical atlas. This draws on the vast neuroendovascular experience of Drs. Adnan H. Siddiqui and J Mocco. The invaluable illustrations by Paul Dressel in the 1st edition of the variations of the vasculature are mostly retained in the 2nd edition. In the 2nd edition, the anatomical photographs are expanded and improved with more modern digital technical aids. Some of the anatomical photographs from the 1st edition have been deleted and replaced with improved versions. As much as possible, color photographs are used, which is an improvement over the 1st edition.

It is my firm belief that the fundamentals of microvascular anatomy and its variations are still the foundation of understanding and practicing any of the disciplines in the clinical neurosciences. Residents and students in neurosurgery, neurology, neuroradiology, and neuroendovascular interventionists should master the neurovascular anatomy as a prerequisite to performing procedures. The time to learn surgical anatomy is not at surgery or during a procedure but in the laboratory. Surgical anatomy is tedious to learn and requires repetition, but when applied clinically, one will rejoice in the knowledge.

In the 2nd edition, I again have attempted to avoid percentages of frequency, preferring to limit the terminology to "frequent," "occasional," and "rare." In addition, there is no exact size of vessels in the illustrations and figures. For this, the 2nd edition again includes the Appendix (1) for relative size of individual vessels depicted in the atlas. Magnification will give different appearances of absolute size, but the relative size of one vessel or structure to another remains the same. It is unusual to measure a vessel at surgery to identify it. Generally, each series of vascular variations is based on at least 20 multiple dissections and, in some cases, on as many as 100 repetitions. No matter how many repetitions are performed, there will always be one more variation.

One must have time, patience, and documentation. Photography is good in certain situations but should be accompanied at least by a basic drawing. There is nothing more frustrating than a high-powered photograph that is incomprehensible without a drawing. Spending time on a detailed drawing and filling in the "gaps" teaches one anatomy at each phase of the learning process (Appendix 2).

Before embarking on the vascular anatomy, one must study the normal background architecture that is the framework of the vasculature of the brain and cranial base.

This involves not just a quick look at the skull or normal brain, but multiple sessions of radiographic and anatomic review of the cranial orifices and sutures, as well as the gyri and sulci of the brain. In the 2nd edition, these fundamental points are shown again in Chapter 1. Magnetic resonance images are not a substitute for viewing real brain or skull specimens.

The 2nd edition retains the principle of focused attention on visualizing the pattern, configuration, and variations of the blood supply. Frequently, a particular branch does not have a name. In certain instances, the complexity and multiplicity of the variations make naming a particular vessel problematic. Many anatomical texts do not take variations into consideration and force a rigid code of naming particular branches of a trunk vessel. Understanding patterns and variations are as important as labeling the particular vessel. The drawings are presented in a fashion that correlates as accurately as possible with an angiographic projection.

The 2nd edition again rests heavily on the wonderful artistic talents of Paul Dressel, who labored diligently to produce the original drawings, as well as the current formatting. Between the 1st and 2nd editions, many additional cadaveric brain dissections were performed by the senior author to confirm and enhance the illustrations of the 1st edition. The extensive dissections on multiple specimens would have not been possible without the support of the Department of Anatomy of the School of Medicine and Biomedical Sciences of the State University of New York at Buffalo, and Dr. Raymond Dannonhoffer, to whom we are very grateful. I am indebted to the assistance and advice of Jody Leonardo, MD, Rabih Tawk, MD, Andrea Chamczuk, MD, Gus Varnavas, MD, Russel Bartels, MD, Natasha Frangopoulos, MD, Jennifer Lin, MD, Alex Mompoint, MD, Josh Meyers, MD, the Buffalo General Foundation, John Tomaszewski, MD (Chairman of the Department of Pathology and Anatomical Sciences, at Buffalo), the Department of Pathology (Buffalo General Hospital), Lucille Miller-Balos, MD (Department of Neuropathology at BGH), Peter Ostrow, MD (Department of Neuropathology at BGH), Reid Heffner, MD (Department of Neuropathology at BGH), Raymond Dannonhoffer, PhD (Administrative Coordinator, Department of Anatomy and Cell Biology at SUNYAB), Leica Microscopes (Larry Bissell), and in memory of Louis Bakay, MD. I am also thankful for the support of the Chairman of the Department of Neurosurgery, Elad I. Levy, MD.

*Walter Grand, MD*
*Senior Author*

# 1 Basic Anatomy

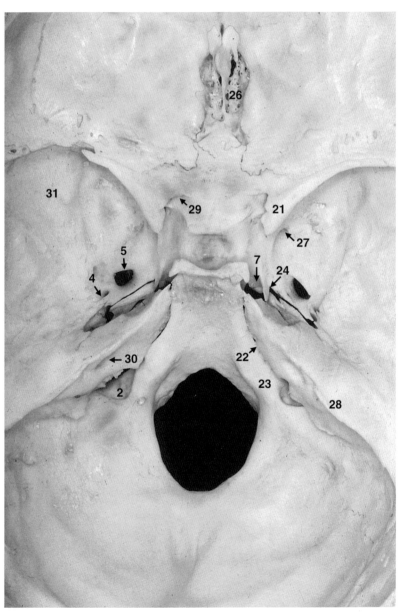

**Fig. 1.1** Interior ventral view of the skull.

2 jugular foramen (bulb)
4 foramen spinosum
5 foramen ovale
7 foramen lacerum
21 anterior clinoid
22 petro-occipital fissure
23 jugular protuberance
24 lingula process
26 cribiform plate
27 foramen rotundum
28 petrous bone
29 optic foramen
30 internal auditory canal
31 temporal fossa

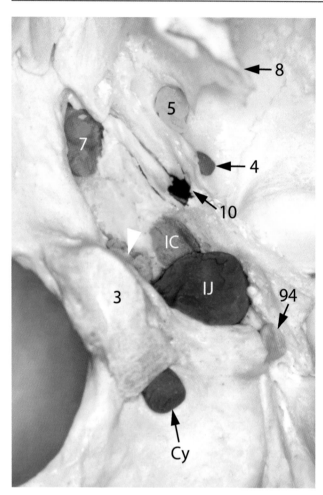

**Fig. 1.2** Ventral view of the left side of the skull base.

IJ  internal jugular vein
IC  internal carotid artery
Cy  condyloid venous foramen
7  foramen lacerum
5  foramen ovale with V3
4  foramen spinosum (middle meningeal artery)
8  lateral pterygoid plate
3  occipital condyle
94  stylomastoid foramen (nerve VII)
10  bony eustachian tube
Arrow  IX, X, XI nerve complex at jugular neural foramen

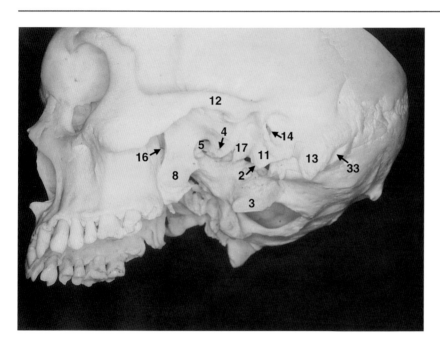

**Fig. 1.3** **(a)** Inferior and lateral view of the skull.

2 jugular foramen (bulb)
3 occipital condyle
4 foramen spinosum
5 foramen ovale
8 lateral pterygoid
11 tympanic plate
12 zygomatic process
13 mastoid process
14 external auditory canal
16 pterygopalatine fossa
17 crista tympanic
33 hypoglossal foramen (nerve XII)

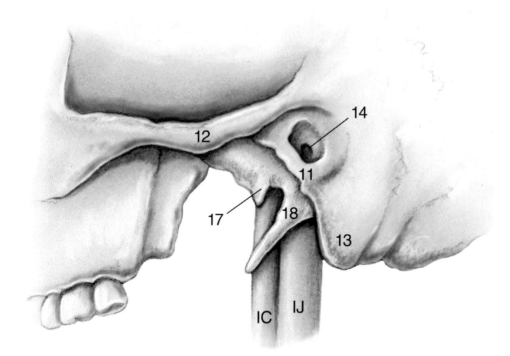

**Fig. 1.3** **(b)** Lateral view of the left cranial base showing the relationship of the styloid process to the internal carotid artery and the internal jugular vein.

11 tympanic plate
12 zygomatic process
13 mastoid process
14 external auditory canal
17 crista tympanic
18 styloid process
IC internal carotid artery
IJ internal jugular vein

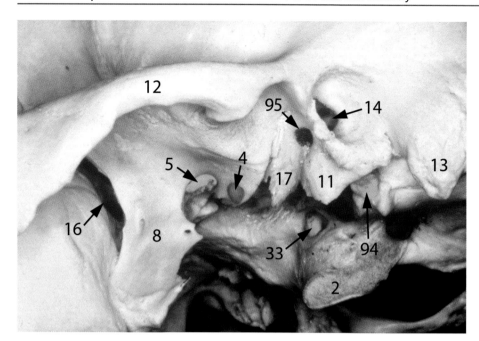

**Fig. 1.4** Lateral view of the left side of the base of the skull.

2   occipital condyle
4   foramen spinosum (middle meningeal artery)
5   foramen ovale (mandibular nerve, V3)
8   lateral pterygoid plate
11  tympanic plate
12  zygomatic process
13  mastoid process
14  external auditory canal
16  pterygopalantine fossa
17  crista tympanic
33  hypoglossal foramen (nerve XII)
94  stylomastoid foramen (nerve VII)
95  surface outline of tympanic cavity

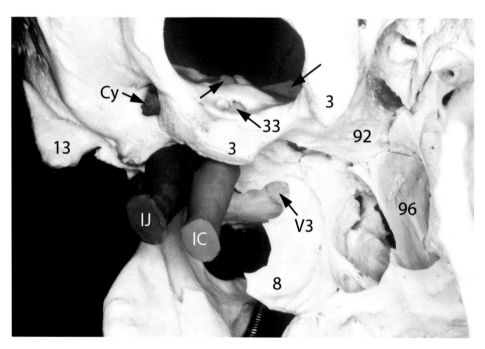

**Fig. 1.5** Ventral-medial view of left skull base.

IJ   internal jugular vein
IC   internal carotid artery
Cy  condyloid emissary vein
V3  mandibular nerve
33  hypoglossal foramen and nerve
8    pterygoid plate
3    occipital condyles; cranial nerves X and XI (*left upper arrow*), trigeminal nerve (*right upper arrow*)
13  left mastoid process
92  clivus
96  vomer

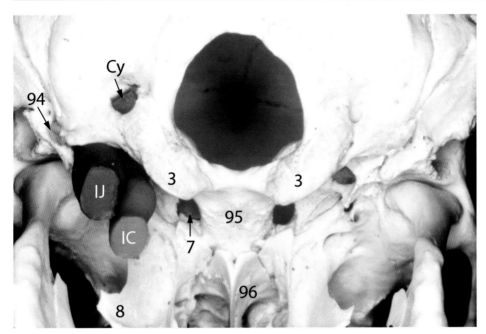

**Fig. 1.6** Ventral view of base of skull.

IC internal carotid artery
IJ internal jugular vein
 7 foramen lacerum
Cy condyloid venous foramen
 3 occipital condyles
95 clivus
96 vomer
 8 lateral pterygoid
94 stylomastoid foramen with cranial nerve VII

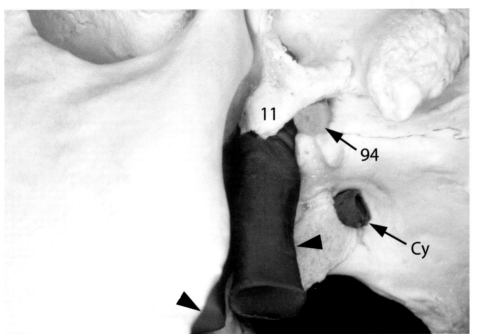

**Fig. 1.7** Lateral view of left side of skull, illustrating relationship of the mandible to the internal jugular vein (*right arrow*) and internal carotid artery (*left arrow*).

Cy condyloid vein
11 tympanic plate
94 stylomastoid foramen with cranial nerve VII

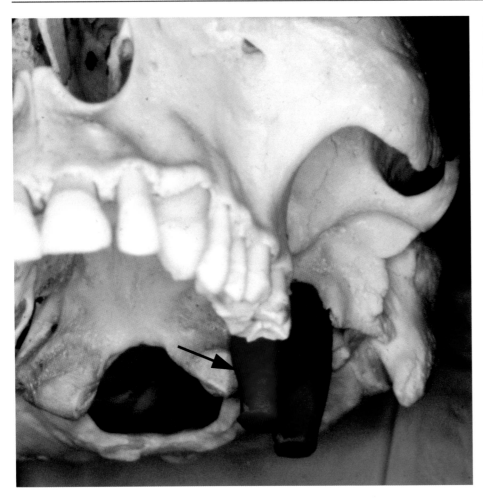

**Fig. 1.8** Anterior-posterior view of relationship of internal carotid artery and internal jugular vein at skull base. Note the medial and anterior position of the internal carotid artery (*arrow*).

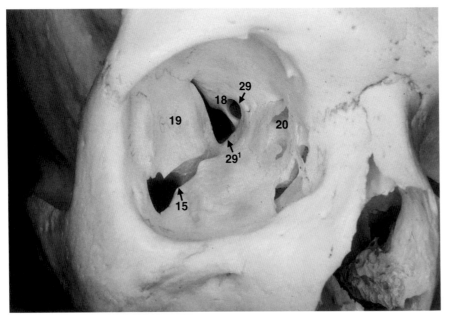

**Fig. 1.9** Oblique view into right orbit.

15  inferior orbital fissure
18  optic strut
19  greater wing of sphenoid
20  ethmoid sinus
29  optic foramen
29[1]  superior orbital fissure

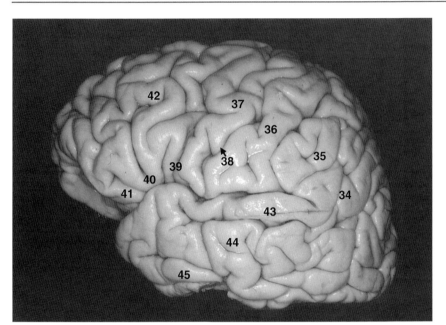

**Fig. 1.10** Lateral view of left hemisphere.

34 angular gyrus
35 supramarginal gyrus
36 postcentral gyrus
37 precentral gyrus
38 central fissure
39 opercularis (inferior frontal gyrus)
40 triangularis (inferior frontal gyrus)
41 orbitalis (inferior frontal gyrus)
42 middle frontal gyrus
43 superior temporal gyrus
44 middle temporal gyrus
45 inferior temporal gyrus

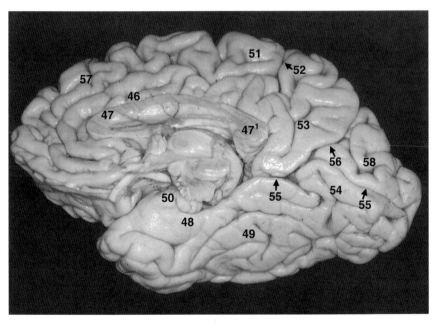

**Fig. 1.11** Infero-medial view of right hemisphere.

46 cingulate gyrus
47 corpus callosum (genu)
47¹ corpus callosum (splenium)
48 parahippocampal gyrus
49 medial occipito-temporal gyrus
50 uncus
51 paracentral lobule
52 marginal ramus (fissure)
53 precuneus
54 lingual gyrus
55 calcarine fissure
56 parieto-occipital fissure
57 medial frontal gyrus
58 cuneus

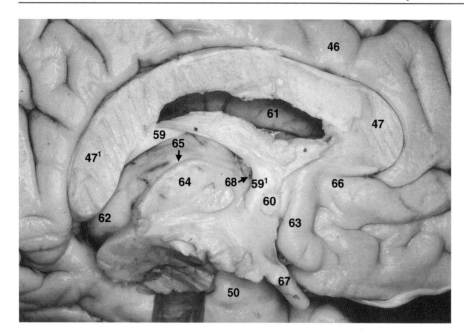

**Fig. 1.12** Close-up medial sagittal view of left hemisphere.

46  cingulate gyrus
47  corpus callosum (genu)
47[1] corpus callosum (splenium)
50  uncus
59  fornix (body)
59[1] fornix (pillar)
60  anterior commissure
61  lateral ventricle
62  pulvinar
63  paraterminal gyrus
64  thalamus (third ventricle)
65  stria medullaris
66  subcallosal (parolfactory area)
67  optic chiasm
68  foramen of monro

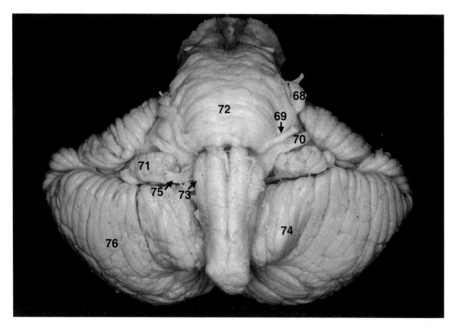

**Fig. 1.13** Ventral view of brain stem and cerebellum.

68  trigeminal nerve (V)
69  facial nerve (VII)
70  vestibulocochlear nerve (VIII)
71  flocculus of cerebellum
72  pons
73  olive
74  tonsil
75  glossopharyngeal nerve (IX)
76  biventral lobule

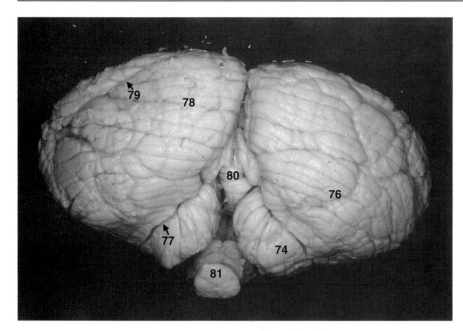

**Fig. 1.14** Infero-posterior view of cerebellum.

74 tonsil
76 biventral lobule
77 retrotonsillar fissure
78 caudal (inferior) semilunar lobule
79 horizontal fissure
80 (inferior) vermis
81 medulla

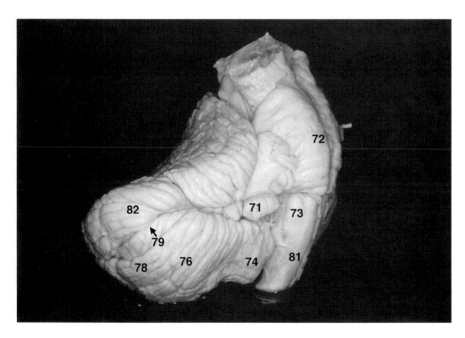

**Fig. 1.15** Lateral-oblique view of right cerebellar hemisphere and brain stem.

71 flocculus
72 pons
73 olive
74 tonsil
76 biventral lobule
78 caudal (inferior) semilunar lobule
79 horizontal fissure
81 medulla
82 rostral (superior) semilunar lobule

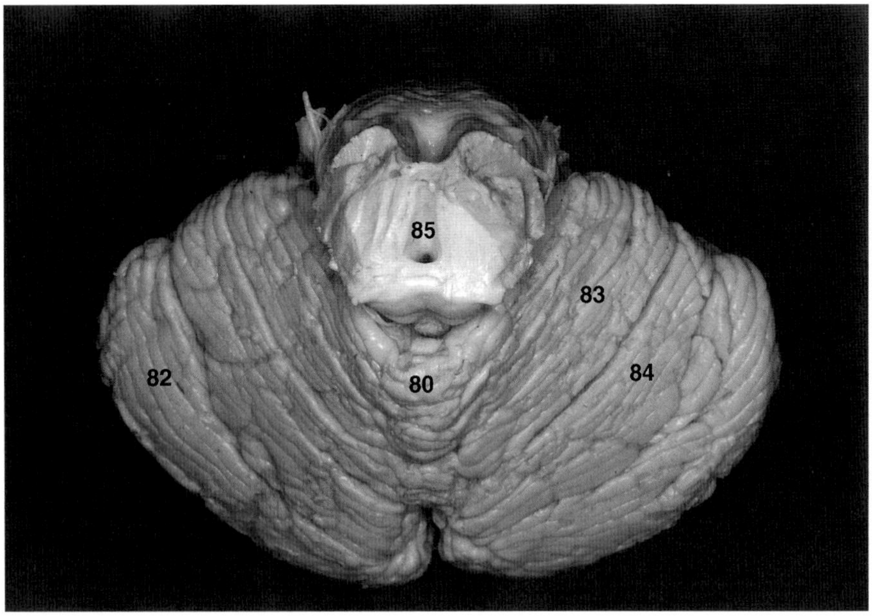

**Fig. 1.16** Superior view of cerebellum.

80 (superior) vermis
82 rostral (superior) semilunar lobule
83 quadrangular lobule
84 simplex lobule
85 aqueduct of Sylvius

# 1.1 Clinical Cases

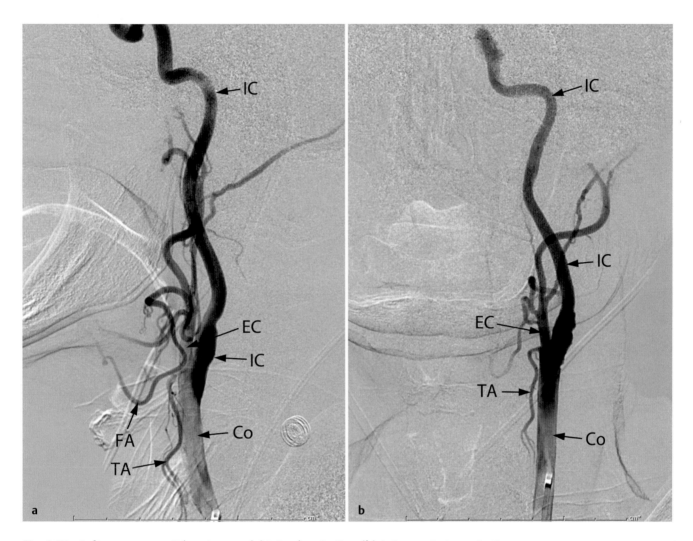

**Fig. 1.17** Left common carotid angiogram. **(a)** Lateral projection. **(b)** Anteroposterior projection.

IC   internal carotid artery
EC   external carotid artery
Co   common carotid artery
FA   facial artery
TA   superior thyroid artery

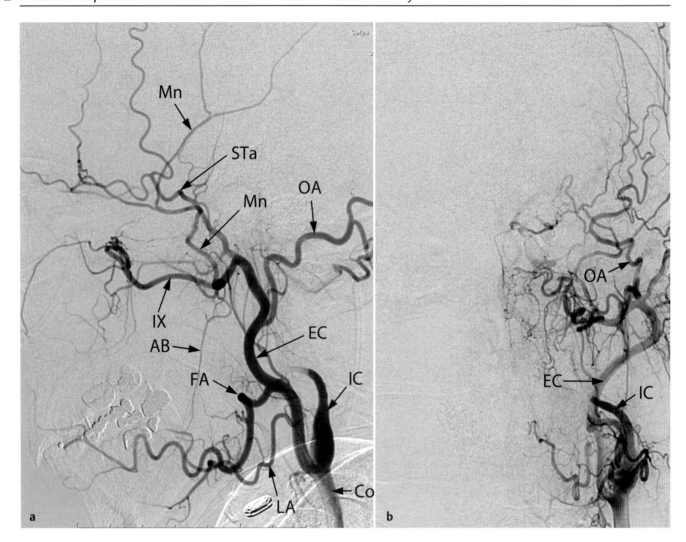

**Fig. 1.18** Left cervical external carotid angiogram. **(a)** Lateral projection. **(b)** Anteroposterior projection.

Mn   middle meningeal artery
STa  superficial temporal artery
OA   occipital artery
IX   internal maxillary artery
AB   buccal artery
EC   external carotid artery
LA   lingual artery
Co   common carotid artery
FA   facial artery
IC   internal carotid artery

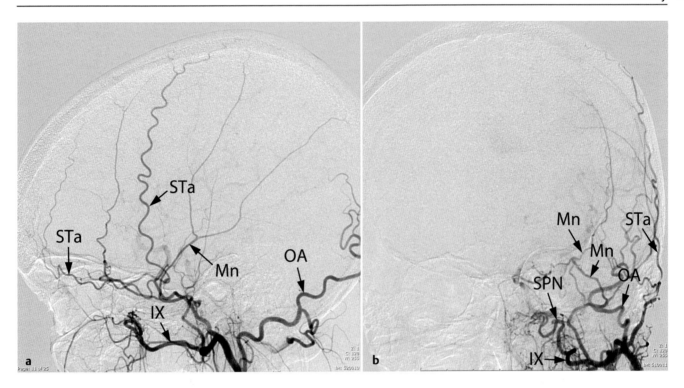

**Fig. 1.19** Left cervical external carotid angiogram. **(a)** Lateral projection. **(b)** Anteroposterior projection.

STa    superficial temporal artery
Mn    middle meningeal artery
OA    occipital artery
IX    internal maxillary artery
SPN    sphenopalatine artery

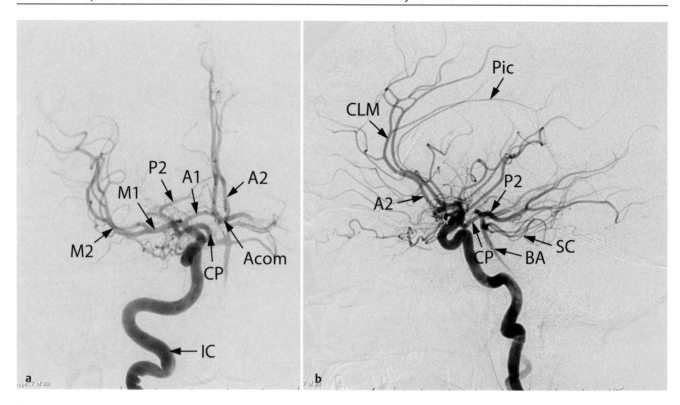

**Fig. 1.20** Right internal carotid artery angiogram. **(a)** Anteroposterior projection. **(b)** Lateral projection.

| | |
|---|---|
| IC | internal carotid artery |
| Acom | anterior communicating artery |
| M1,M2 | middle cerebral artery |
| A1, A2 | anterior cerebral artery |
| CP | posterior communicating artery |
| P2 | posterior cerebral artery |
| Pic | pericallosal artery |
| CLM | callosomarginal artery |
| BA | basilar artery |
| SC | superior cerebellar artery |

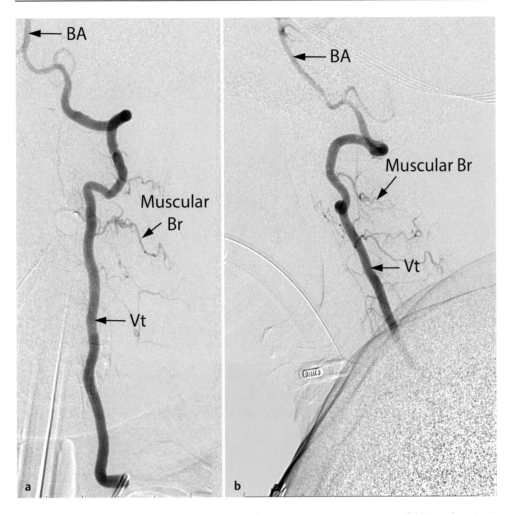

**Fig. 1.21** Left cervical vertebral angiogram. **(a)** Anteroposterior projection. **(b)** Lateral projection.

BA  basilar artery
Vt  vertebral artery
Br  branch

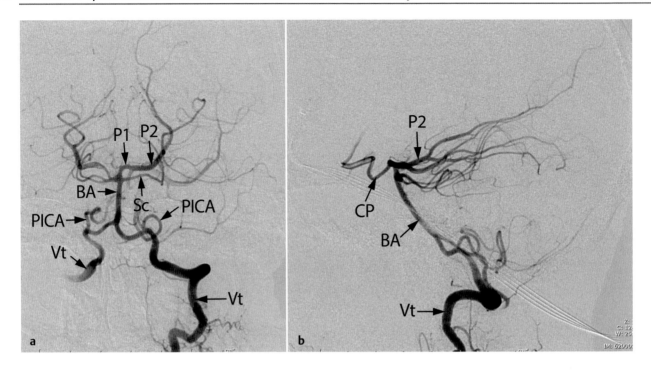

**Fig. 1.22** Left vertebral angiogram of intracranial vessels. **(a)** Anteroposterior projection. **(b)** Lateral projection.

| | |
|---|---|
| BA | basilar artery |
| Vt | vertebral artery |
| Sc | superior cerebellar artery |
| P1, P2 | posterior cerebral artery |
| PICA | posterior inferior cerebellar artery |
| CP | posterior communicating artery |

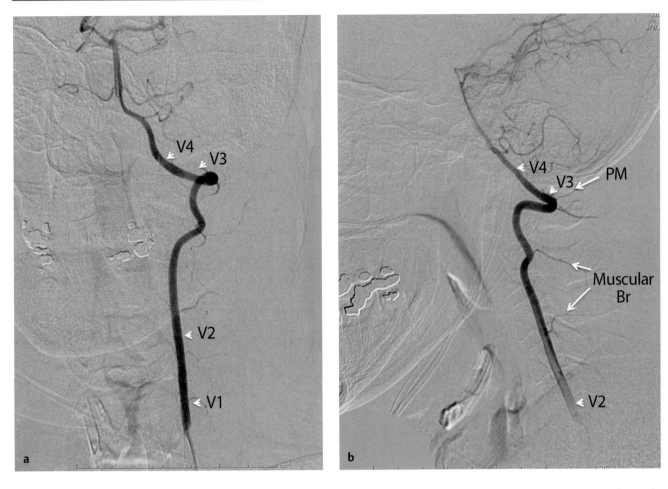

**Fig. 1.23** **(a)** Anteroposterior projection of the left vertebral angiogram emphasizing vertebral artery segments in the neck. **(b)** Lateral projection.

V1   extraosseous
V2   foraminal
V3   extraspinal
V4   intradural
PM   posterior meningeal branch
Br   branch

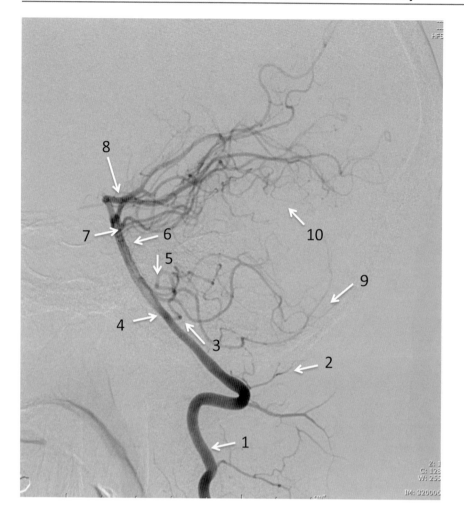

**Fig. 1.24** Lateral left vertebral angiogram focused on intracranial branches.

1   vertebral artery
2   posterior meningeal artery
3   posterior inferior cerebellar artery
4   basilar artery
5   anterior inferior cerebellar artery
6   lateral pontine branches
7   superior cerebellar artery
8   posterior cerebral artery
9   cerebellar hemispheric branches in the great horizontal fissure
10   superior cerebellar artery branches

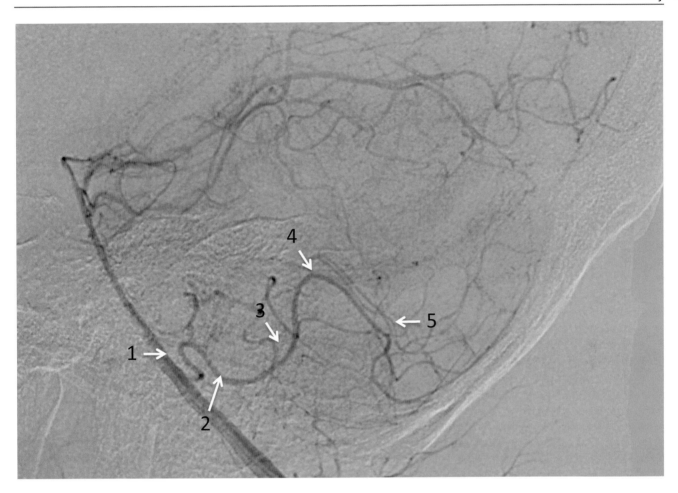

**Fig. 1.25** Lateral left vertebral intracranial angiogram.

1   anterior medullary segment of posterior inferior cerebellar artery (PICA)
2   lateral medullary segment (PICA)
3   posterior medullary segment (PICA)
4   supra-tonsillar segment (PICA)
5   hemispheric and vermian branches (PICA)

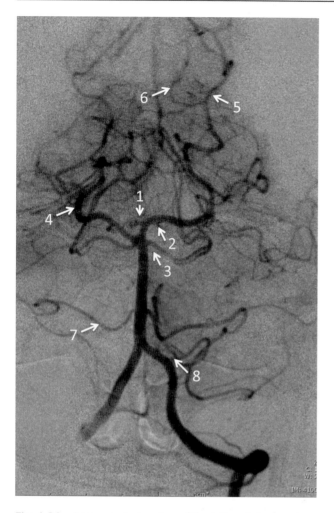

**Fig. 1.26** Anteroposterior view of the left vertebral angiogram.

1    thalamoperforating and thalamogeniculate arteries
2    P1 segment of the posterior cerebral artery
3    superior cerebellar artery
4    P2 ambient segment of the posterior cerebral artery
5    parieto-occipital artery
6    calcarine artery
7    anterior inferior cerebellar artery
8    posterior inferior cerebellar artery

# 2 External Carotid Artery

At its origin from the common carotid artery in the neck, the external carotid artery can be found in a triangular space with the sternocleidomastoid muscle posteriorly, the omohyoid muscle inferiorly, and the posterior belly of the digastric muscle and stylohyoid muscle superiorly. The external carotid artery passes medial to the posterior belly of the digastric and stylohyoid muscles. It terminates posterior to the neck of the mandible, where it divides into the internal maxillary and superficial temporal arteries. The internal maxillary artery then passes medial to the mandible into the subtemporal fossa. The superficial temporal artery continues anterior to the tragus of the ear and over the zygomatic bone.

Branching of the external carotid artery is classified into two components, the first being the more proximal branches from the main stem of the external carotid artery, and the other the terminal branches from the internal maxillary artery and the superficial temporal artery.

## 2.1 Proximal Branches of the External Carotid Artery

### 2.1.1 Superior Thyroid Artery

This is the first branch of the external carotid artery. It originates opposite the level of the hyoid bone and passes to the upper portion of the thyroid gland.

### 2.1.2 Lingual Artery

The lingual artery arises from the external carotid artery just above the superior thyroid artery. The first part of the lingual artery is crossed by the hypoglossal nerve as it passes into the musculature of the tongue.

### 2.1.3 Facial Artery

The facial artery usually arises from the external carotid artery a few millimeters above the origin of the lingual artery and, at times, may almost have a common origin with the lingual artery. It courses deep to the posterior belly of the digastric and stylohyoid muscles and then runs in a groove along the lower jaw, passing above the jaw into the cheek. It terminates at the inner canthus of the eye as the angular artery. The angular artery is an important collateralization with the ophthalmic artery distribution as an alternative retrograde blood supply to the internal carotid artery system. Close to its origin, the facial artery gives off the ascending palatine artery, which passes to the tonsils and the eustachian tube.

Despite the description in many texts of a bifurcation of the external carotid artery into the superficial temporal artery and internal maxillary artery, on occasion, the external carotid artery has a major bifurcation after the facial artery, with a posterior branch becoming the occipital artery and, at times, an occipital artery–ascending pharyngeal complex. The ascending pharyngeal and occipital arteries have a variable relationship not only to each other but also to the main stem of the external carotid artery.

### 2.1.4 Occipital Artery

The occipital artery arises from the posterior wall of the external carotid artery and crosses the internal carotid artery. The hypoglossal nerve crosses it inferiorly close to its origin. The occipital artery then courses in the interval between the transverse process of the atlas and the mastoid tip and has a sinuous course over the occiput. Its distal branches are somewhat variable, but it may give off a posterior meningeal branch that ascends through the jugular foramen to supply the dura of the posterior fossa. The most important muscular branch is the sternomastoid branch, which usually arises early in the course of the occipital artery and can loop downward across the hypoglossal nerve before entering the sternomastoid muscle. Just above and behind the mastoid, the occipital artery usually gives off a penetrating mastoid artery that pierces the skull through a foramen to supply the dura of the posterior fossa as well. The occipital artery supplies numerous branches to the musculature in the suboccipital region, which anastomose with the muscular branches of the vertebral artery. This can, on occasion, lead to "dangerous anastomoses" with the vertebral artery.

### 2.1.5 Posterior Auricular Artery

The posterior auricular artery usually originates from the external carotid artery distal to the origin of the occipital artery, but it may arise from the occipital artery itself. It terminates at the space between the external auditory meatus and the mastoid process. The stylomastoid branch at the lower external meatus enters the stylomastoid foramen alongside the facial nerve.

### 2.1.6 Ascending Pharyngeal Artery

The ascending pharyngeal artery frequently originates from the back of the external carotid artery near the bifurcation of the common carotid artery. However, its origin and configuration can be quite variable. It may originate from the internal carotid artery, from the base of the occipital artery, or more distally on the occipital artery. As the ascending pharyngeal artery moves superiorly, it gives off muscular branches to the pharynx and supplies the eustachian tube. Prior to the branches to the eustachian tube, the ascending pharyngeal artery may give off a posterior meningeal branch that either ascends through the jugular foramen, along with the tenth and eleventh nerve, or through the hypoglossal foramen in proximity to the hypoglossal nerve. At times, the posterior meningeal artery arising from the ascending pharyngeal artery can bifurcate, giving branches to the posterior fossa dura through both the hypoglossal foramen and the jugular foramen. The ascending pharyngeal artery may also form dangerous anastomoses with the ipsilateral vertebral artery.

## 2.2 Distal Branches of the External Carotid Artery

### 2.2.1 Superficial Temporal Artery

The superficial temporal artery originates in the substance of the parotid gland, at the back of the base of the mandible, as one division of the terminal bifurcation of the external carotid artery. At times, it appears to originate as a lesser branch of the external carotid artery. It courses above the zygomatic arch and branches into anterior and posterior divisions. The transverse facial branch originates at the anterior border of the parotid gland and runs anteriorly, accompanied by the buccal or zygomatic branches of the facial nerve.

### 2.2.2 Internal Maxillary Artery

The internal maxillary artery is the main continuation of the external carotid artery. Initially, it is embedded in the parotid gland and passes behind the ramus of the mandible, covering the surface of the lateral pterygoid muscles. The internal maxillary artery, in its subtemporal course, can lie deep to or superficial to the lateral pterygoid muscle. In the former case, the buccal branch of the third division of the fifth nerve passes over the internal maxillary artery as it courses past the foramen ovale, whereas the remainder of the third division of the fifth nerve passes medial to the internal maxillary artery. The middle meningeal artery arises from the internal maxillary artery to pass through the foramen spinosum, and two roots of the auricular temporal nerve pass on either side of the artery. The buccal arterial branch runs with the buccal nerve as the nerve branches from the third division of the fifth nerve. Frequently, the internal maxillary artery gives off an accessory meningeal artery that runs directly through the foramen ovale. At times, the accessory meningeal artery can originate from the middle meningeal artery itself. As the internal maxillary artery courses more distally and anteriorly, it gives off deep temporal branches to the temporalis muscle.

As the internal maxillary artery approaches the sphenopalatine fossa anterior to the lateral pterygoid plate, it distributes the posterior-superior alveolar artery over the maxillary bone. The internal maxillary artery then passes deep to the lateral pterygoid plate to enter the sphenopalatine fossa. It supplies a branch, the infraorbital artery, which runs inferior to the second division of the fifth nerve as they both enter the infraorbital canal. At the base of the proximal infraorbital artery, the sphenopalatine branch arises and courses through the sphenopalatine foramen into the nasal cavity as the terminal branch of the internal maxillary artery.

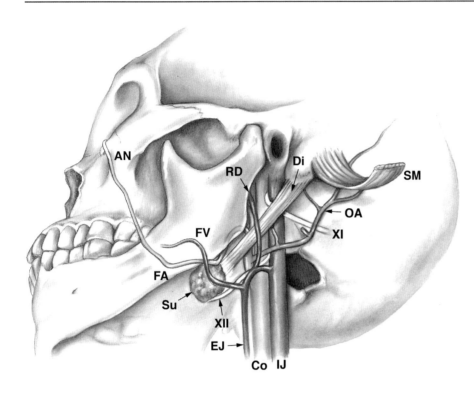

**Fig. 2.1** Superficial neck and retro-mandibular region.

Su  submandibular gland
XI  eleventh nerve
XII  twelfth nerve (hypoglossal)
SM  sternocleidomastoid muscle
AN  angular artery
Di  posterior belly diagastric muscle
EJ  external jugular vein
FV  facial vein
FA  facial artery
Co  common carotid artery
IJ  internal jugular vein
OA  occipital artery
RD  retromandibular vein

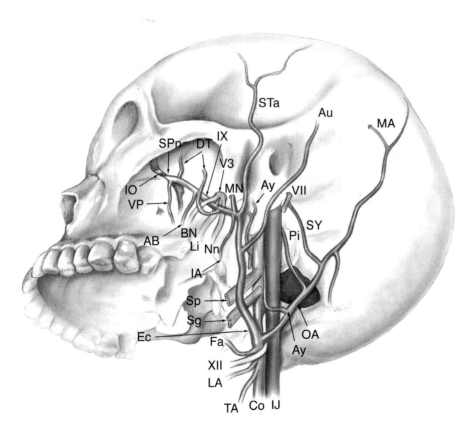

**Fig. 2.2** Deep anatomy with removal of mandible and exposure of subtemporal fossa and extensive branches of the internal maxillary artery.

AB  buccal artery
Au  posterior auricular artery
Ay  ascending pharyngeal artery
BN  buccal nerve
Co  common carotid artery
DT  deep temporal arteries
Ec  external carotid artery
Fa  facial artery
IO  infraorbital nerve (V2)
IA  inferior alveolar artery
IJ  internal jugular vein
IX  internal maxillary artery
Li  lingual nerve
LA  lingual artery
MA  mastoid artery
MN  middle meningeal artery
Nn  inferior alveolar nerve
OA  occipital artery
Pi  posterior meningeal artery
Sg  styloglossus muscle
Sp  stylopharyngeus muscle
SPn  sphenopalatine artery
STa  superficial temporal artery
SY  stylomastoid artery
TA  superior thyroid artery
VP  posterior superior alveolar artery
VII  seventh nerve
XII  twelfth nerve (hypoglossal)
V3  third division fifth nerve

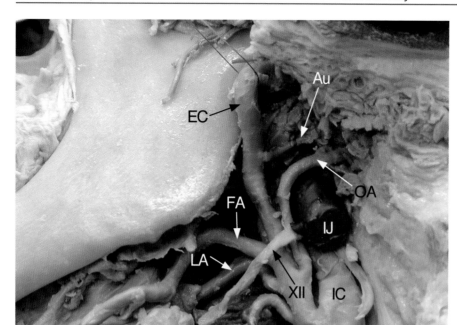

**Fig. 2.3** Submandibular view of the carotid complex.

IJ internal jugular vein
XII hypoglossal nerve
FA facial artery
LA lingual artery
TA superior thyroid artery
Au posterior auricular artery
OA occipital artery
EC external carotid artery
IC internal carotid artery

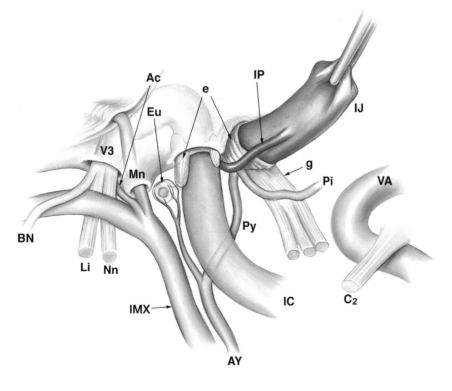

**Fig. 2.4** Lateral close-up view of left subtemporal fossa. Note inferior petrosal vein (IP) joining internal jugular vein in neck.

Ac accessory meningeal artery
AY ascending pharyngeal artery
BN buccal nerve
$C_2$ second cervical nerve
Eu eustachian tube
IC internal carotid artery
IP inferior petrosal vein
IJ internal jugular vein
IMX internal maxillary artery
Li lingual nerve
Mn middle meningeal artery
Nn inferior alveolar nerve
Pi posterior meningeal artery (occipital)
Py posterior meningeal artery (ascending pharyngeal)
VA vertebral artery
V3 third division of fifth nerve
e fibrous band
g pars nervosa

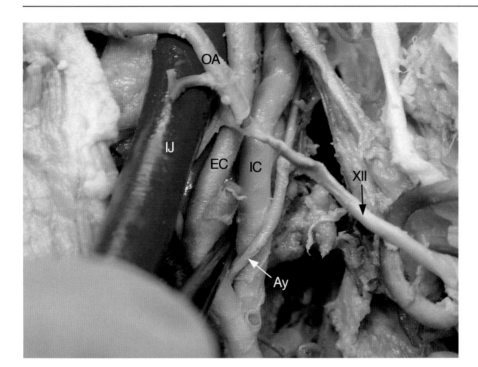

**Fig. 2.5** Right side of neck. Ascending pharyngeal artery (Ay) arising from base of the external carotid artery (EC).

IC internal carotid artery
XII hypoglossal nerve
OA occipital artery
IJ internal jugular vein

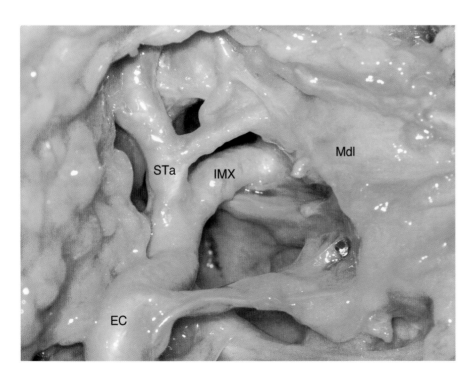

**Fig. 2.6** The external carotid artery (EC) on the right bifurcating into the superficial temporal artery (STa) and the internal maxillary artery (IMX), as the IMX disappears behind the angle of the mandible (Mdl) into the subtemporal fossa.

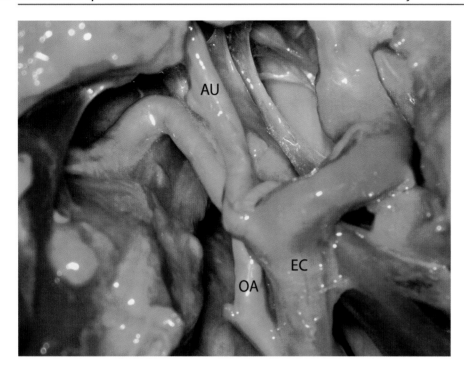

**Fig. 2.7** The occipital artery (OA) and the posterior auricular artery (AU) branching off from the external carotid artery (EC) on the right side.

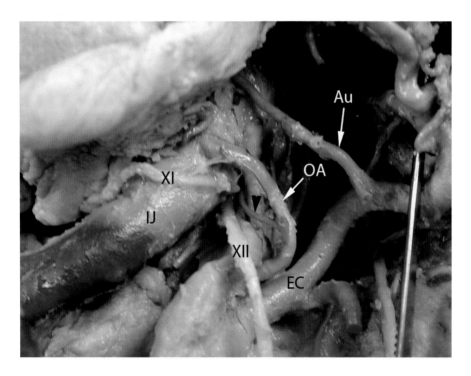

**Fig. 2.8** The eleventh nerve (XI) passes deep to the internal jugular vein (IJ) and then turns posteriorly, superficial to the IJ.

XII    hypoglossal nerve
OA    occipital artery
Au    posterior auricular artery
EC    external carotid artery
Arrowhead    branch of OA to jugular
            foramen to supply
            posterior fossa dura

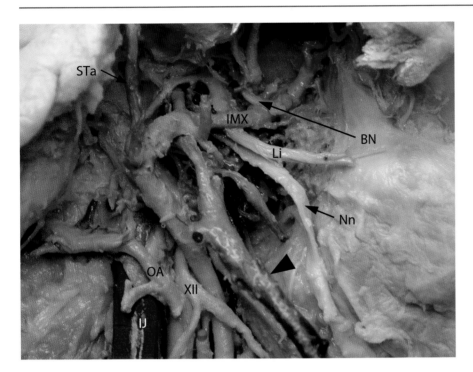

**Fig. 2.9** Internal maxillary artery (IMX) coursing in subtemporal fossa on the right. Both the lingual nerve (Li) and the inferior alveolar nerve (Nn) pass medial to the IMX.

BN   buccal nerve
STa  superficial temporal artery
OA   occipital artery
IJ   internal jugular vein
XII  hypoglossal nerve
Arrowhead   a large vein draining the subtemporal fossa and joined to the common facial vein (*not shown*)

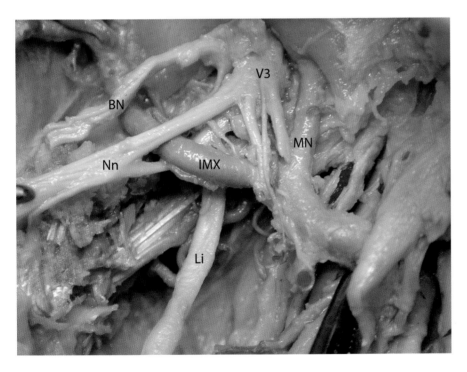

**Fig. 2.10** Left side. The internal maxillary artery (IMX) pierces the inferior alveolar nerve (Nn).

BN   buccal nerve
Li   lingual nerve
V3   mandibular nerve
MN   middle meningeal artery

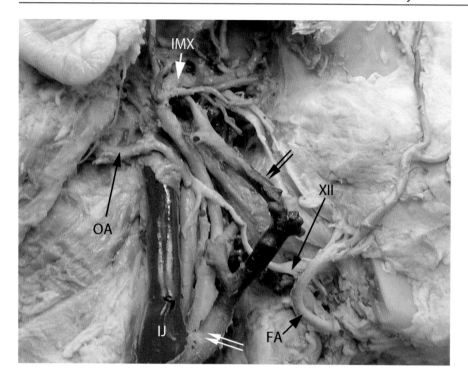

**Fig. 2.11** Right common facial vein (*white double arrows*) joining internal jugular vein (IJ). There is a large vein from the subtemporal fossa (*black double arrows*) as a tributary to the common facial vein.

FA   facial artery
IMX internal maxillary artery
OA   occipital artery
XII   hypoglossal nerve

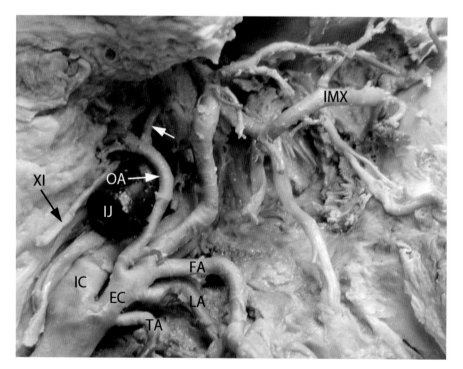

**Fig. 2.12** The right occipital artery (OA) gives a branch (*arrow*) to the posterior fossa dura through the jugular foramen. The eleventh nerve (XI) has passed medial and posterior to the internal jugular vein (IJ).

FA   facial artery
LA   lingual artery
TA   superior thyroid artery
IMX internal maxillary artery
IC   internal carotid artery
EC   external carotid artery

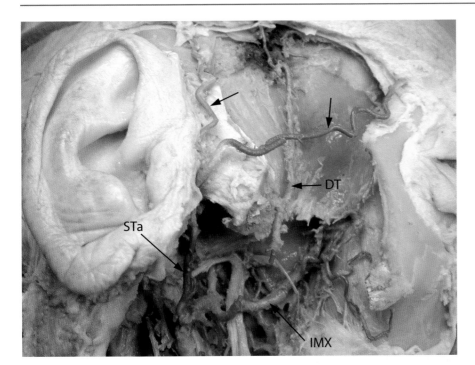

**Fig. 2.13** Bifurcation of the superficial temporal artery (STa) into posterior (*left arrow*) and anterior (*right arrow*) branches in the subgaleal plane. A branch to the temporalis muscle (DT) from the internal maxillary artery (IMX) passes deep to the STa.

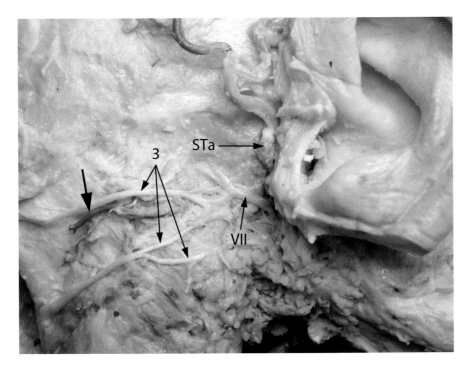

**2.14** Relationship of the emergence of the seventh nerve (VII) to the root of the superficial temporal artery (STa).

3 Buccal branches of VII nerve
Arrow transfacial artery

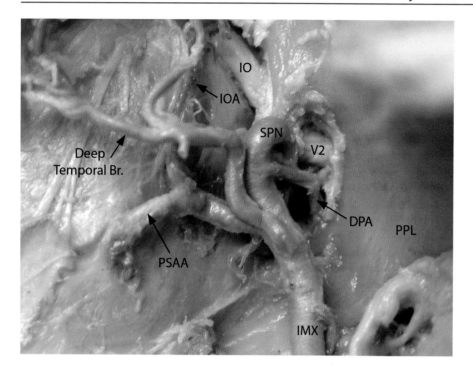

**2.15** Termination of the internal maxillary artery (IMX) at the sphenopalatine fossa in front of the pterygoid plate (PPL). (V2) Second division of the fifth nerve transitioning into the infraorbital nerve (IO).

SPN   sphenopalatine artery
IOA   infraorbital artery
PSAA  posterior inferior alveolar artery
DPA   descending palatine artery

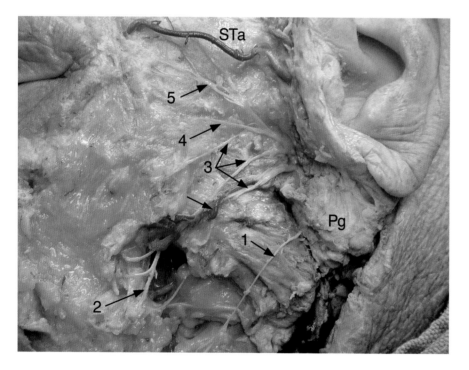

**Fig. 2.16** Left side of face. Dissection of facial nerve in relationship to transfacial artery (*arrow*) and anterior branch of the superficial temporal artery (STa).

1   cervical branch
2   mandibular branch
3   buccal branches
4   zygomatic branch
5   temporo-zygomatic branch
Pg  parotid gland

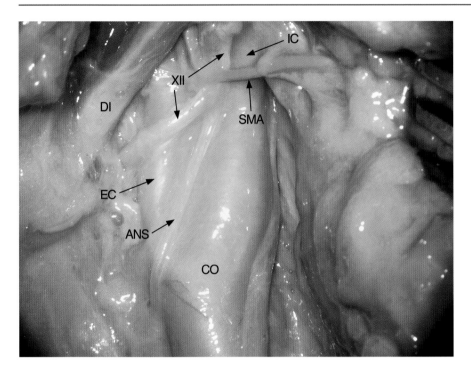

**Fig. 2.17** Exposure of the left common carotid artery (CO) in the neck, illustrating the hypoglossal nerve (XII) looping under an arterial branch to the sternocleidomastoid muscle from the external carotid artery (EC).

DI    posterior belly of digastric muscle
ANS   descending ansa-hypoglossus
SMA   artery to sternocleidomastoid muscle
IC    internal carotid artery

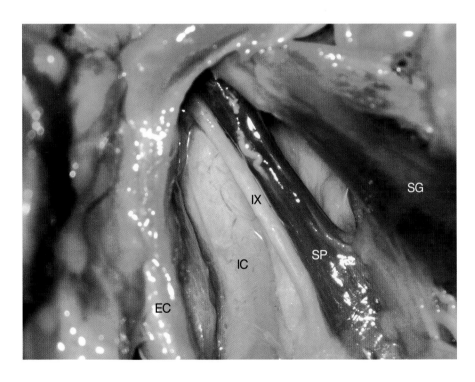

**Fig. 2.18** Right internal carotid artery (IC) with nerve IX crossing obliquely and into the pharyngeal constrictors.

SP    stylopharyngeous muscle
SG    styloglossus muscle
EC    external carotid artery

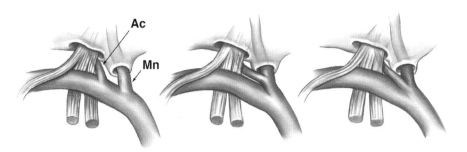

**Fig. 2.19** Left lateral close-up view of origin of middle meningeal artery (Mn) and variations of relationship to accessory meningeal artery (Ac).

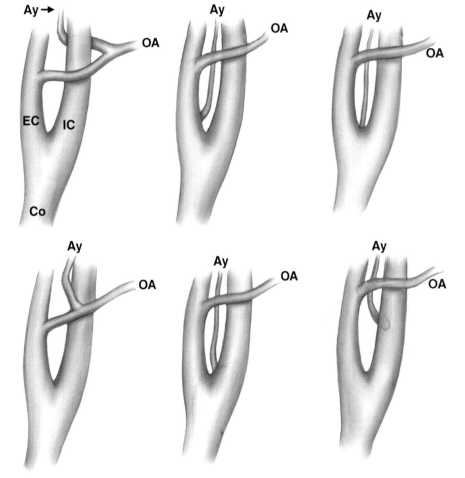

**Fig. 2.20** Variations of ascending pharyngeal origin from common carotid bifurcation.

Ay   ascending pharyngeal artery
Co   common carotid artery
EC   external carotid artery
IC   internal carotid artery
OA   occipital artery

## 2.3  Clinical Cases

### 2.3.1  Case 1

A teenager presented with an increasing, painless swelling in the neck. Magnetic resonance imaging (MRI) revealed a uniformly enhancing mass splaying the carotid bifurcation. An angiogram confirmed a carotid body tumor supplied by multiple branches from the proximal external carotid artery with a robust vascular blush. These branches were selectively catheterized and embolized using a liquid embolic agent after the teenager had passed a carotid balloon test occlusion. The mass was resected through a transcervical incision and preservation of the internal carotid artery. The pathology was consistent with a benign carotid body glomus tumor.

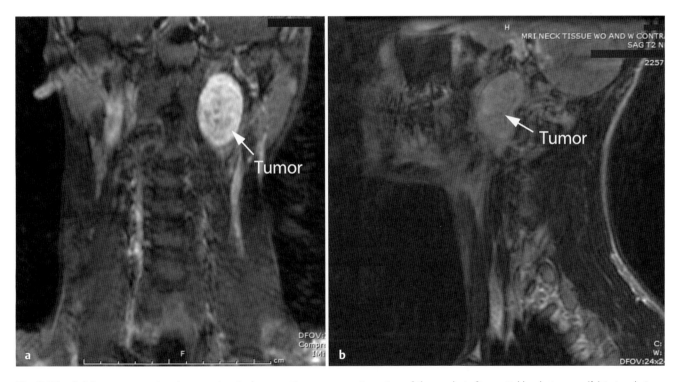

**Fig. 2.21**   (a) Anteroposterior view, contrasted magnetic resonance imaging of the neck. Left carotid body tumor. (b) Lateral view.

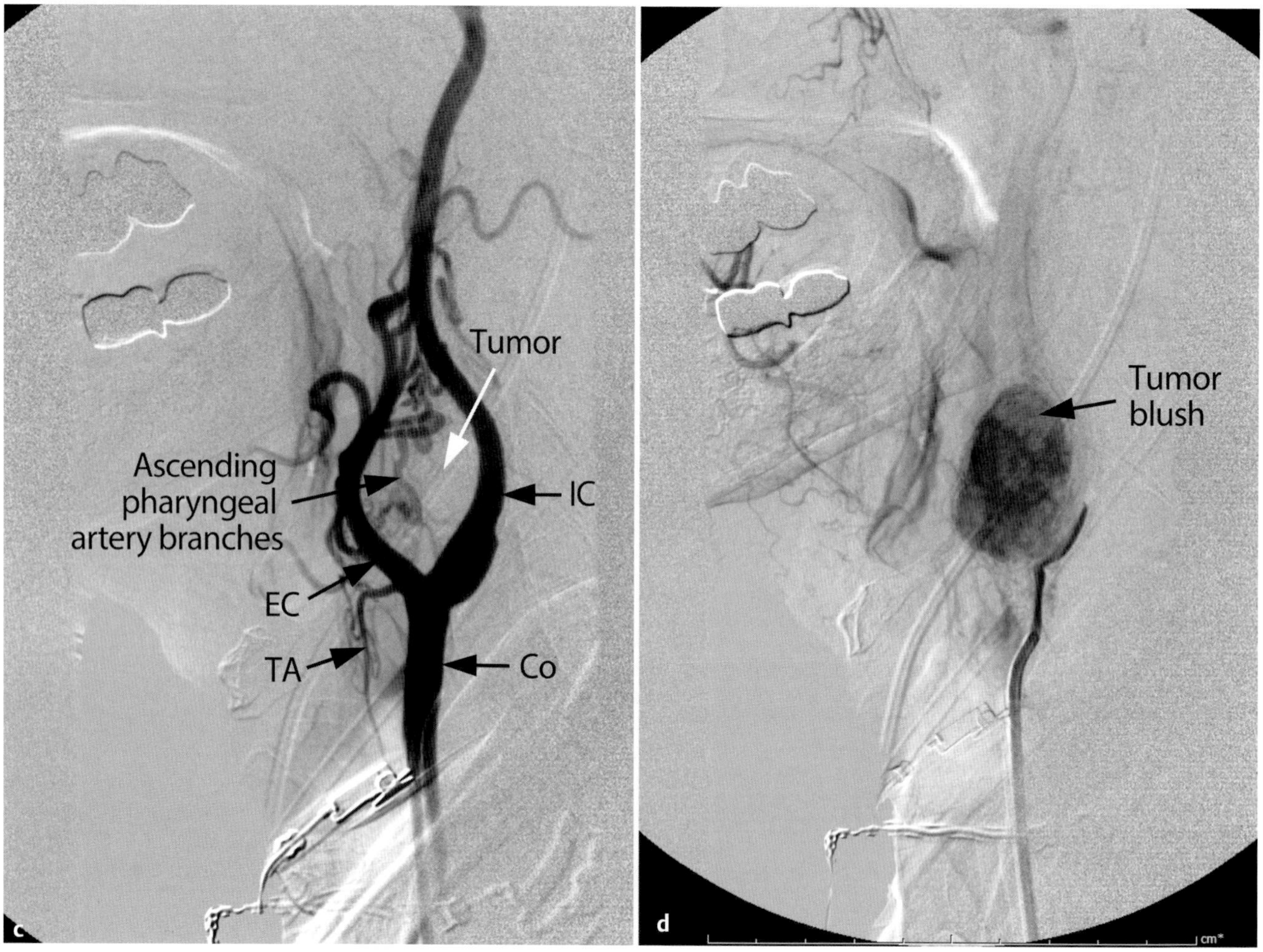

**Fig. 2.21** (*Continued*) **(c)** Left common carotid (Co) angiogram. Splaying of the internal carotid (IC) and external carotid (EC) arteries by the tumor. Superior thyroid artery (TA); ascending pharyngeal artery branches (*arrow*). **(d)** Late phase with tumor blush.

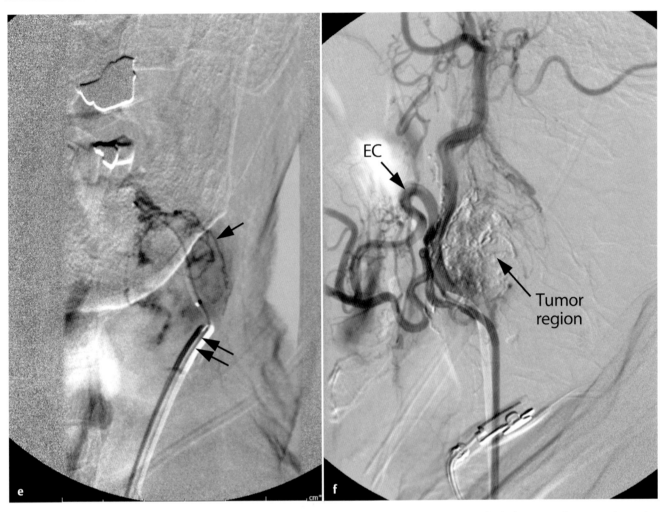

**Fig. 2.21** (*Continued*)  **(e)** Microcatheterization (*double arrows*) of the external carotid artery (EC) shows a robust supply to the tumor (*arrow*). **(f)** Postembolization with delayed-phase cervical angiogram shows preservation of the EC artery branches and no vascular tumor blush.

## 2.3.2 Case 2

A middle-aged woman presented with personality changes and increasing headaches that would awaken her. MRI revealed a large right frontal convexity dural-based mass with tremendous cerebral edema in the subjacent right frontal cortex. An angiogram confirmed a prominent vascular supply from the right middle meningeal artery, which was embolized using liquid embolics. The tumor was removed through a right frontal craniotomy. Pathology was consistent with a benign meningioma.

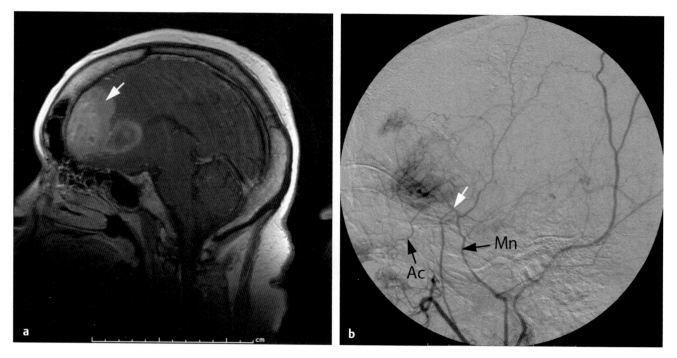

**Fig. 2.22** **(a)** A sagittal T1 contrasted magnetic resonance image of the brain. There is a large, heterogeneous, enhancing, partially cystic, dural-based mass (*arrow*). There is surrounding edema. **(b)** A selective left external carotid angiogram shows a prominent supply to the mass from the frontal branch (*arrow*) of the middle meningeal artery (Mn) and contribution from the accessory meningeal artery (Ac).

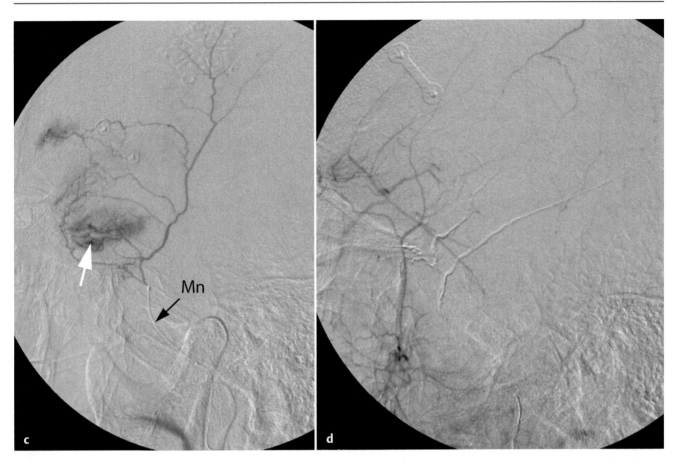

**Fig. 2.22** (*Continued*)    **(c)** Microcatheter in the middle meningeal artery (Mn). There is a tumor blush from the Mn (*white arrow*). **(d)** Post–liquid embolization through the Mn with removal of the tumor blush.

### 2.3.3 Case 3

A 12-year-old boy presented with a syncopal event and rapidly increasing right-sided facial swelling. MRI revealed a posterior, nasopharyngeal, uniformly enhancing mass with prominent flow voids extending into the maxillary sinus anteroinferiorly, the right orbit, and the ethmoid and sphenoid sinuses. Computed tomography (CT) confirmed erosion and remodeling of bone. Angiography revealed a prominent vascular supply from the terminal external carotid artery branches of the internal maxillary artery, including the middle meningeal, accessory meningeal, sphenopalatine, and ethmoidal branches. In addition, there was contribution from the cavernous branches of the internal carotid artery, primarily the inferolateral trunk. The sphenopalatine and accessory meningeal arteries were embolized. A prominent connection was noted between the middle meningeal artery (Mn) and the ophthalmic artery through the recurrent meningeal artery, which was first coiled, and then the Mn was embolized to protect embolic material from flowing into the ophthalmic or internal carotid artery. Postembolization the tumor was removed through an extended endonasal transmaxillary approach. The patient made an excellent recovery without any deficits. The pathology was consistent with juvenile nasal angiofibroma.

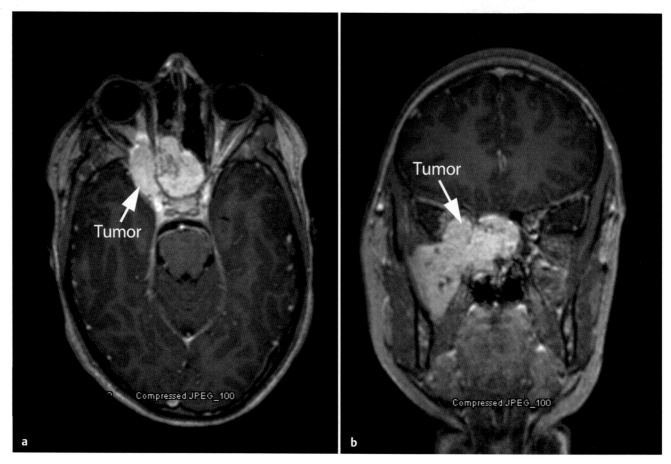

**Fig. 2.23** **(a)** Horizontal section of T1 contrasted magnetic resonance imaging of the skull base. There is an enhancing mass in the nasopharynx and skull base. **(b)** Coronal section.

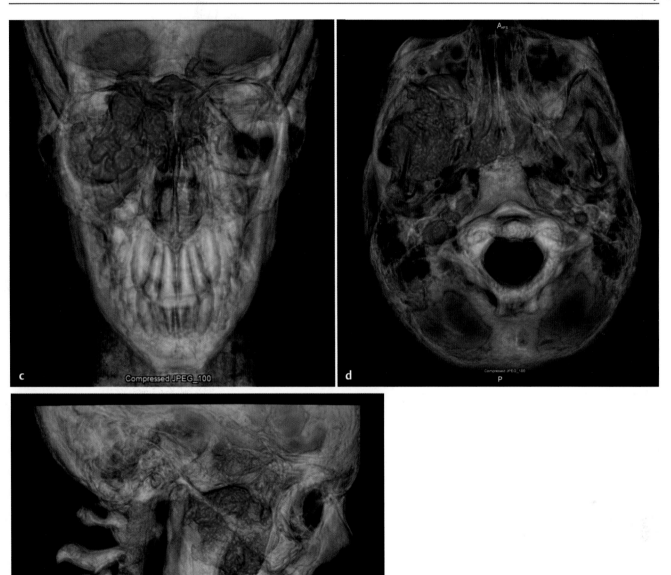

**Fig. 2.23** (*Continued*) **(c)** Coronal three-dimensional computed tomographic reconstruction of the skull base showing the tumor's relationship to the bony structures of the skull. **(d)** Horizontal section. **(e)** Lateral view.

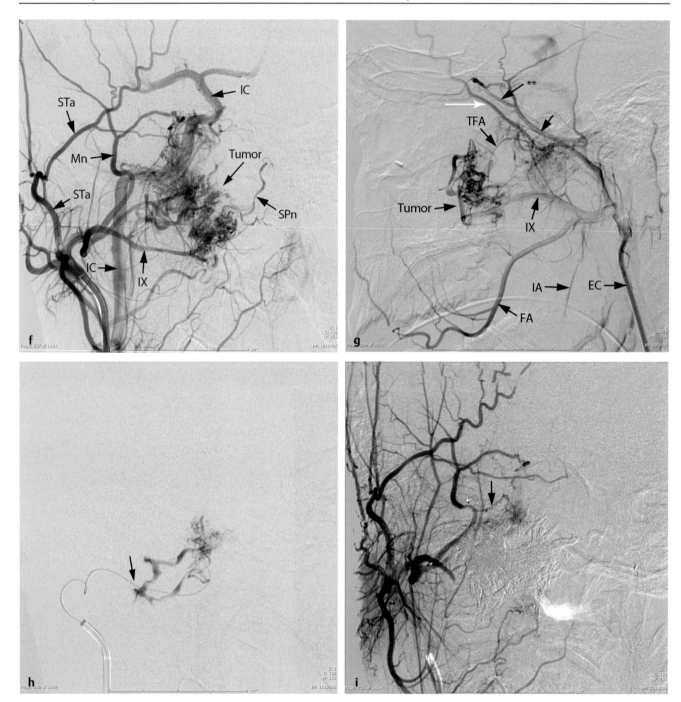

**Fig. 2.23** (*Continued*)  **(f)** Anteroposterior view of a selective microcatheter angiogram of the external carotid artery. Mn, middle meningeal artery; SPn, sphenopalatine artery; STa, superficial temporal artery; IX, internal maxillary artery; IC, internal carotid artery. **(g)** Lateral view of **(f)**. FA, facial artery; EC, external carotid artery; IX, internal maxillary artery; IA, inferior alveolar artery; Mn, middle meningeal artery. *\*\**, recurrent meningeal branch of Mn (*upper arrows*); DTA, deep temporal artery (*white arrow*); TFA, transverse facial artery. **(h)** Selective embolization with onyx of the branches of the internal maxillary artery at the sphenopalatine junction (*arrow*). **(i)** Postembolization external carotid angiogram. There are residual feeding vessels (*arrow*) to the tumor from the middle meningeal artery.

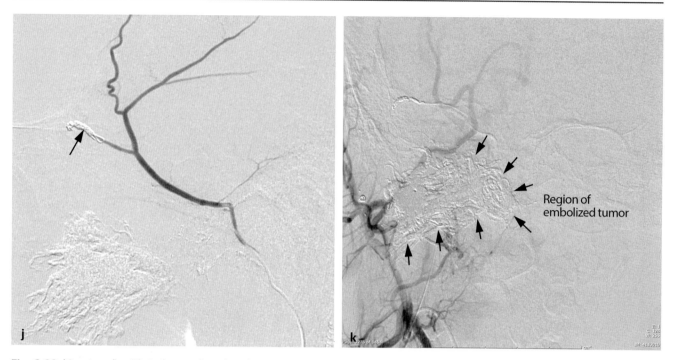

**Fig. 2.23** (*Continued*)  **(j)** Coils are placed in the middle meningeal branch (*arrow*). **(k)** Embolization completed with no tumor blush.

## Clinical Pearls

- The angular artery is an important collateralization with the ophthalmic artery distribution as an alternative retrograde blood supply to the internal carotid artery system.

- Just above and behind the mastoid, the occipital artery usually gives off a penetrating mastoid artery that pierces the skull through a foramen to supply the dura of the posterior fossa as well. The occipital artery supplies numerous branches to the musculature in the suboccipital region, which anastomose with the muscular branches of the vertebral artery. This can, on occasion, lead to "dangerous anastomoses" with the vertebral artery.

- The stylomastoid branch at the lower external meatus enters the stylomastoid foramen alongside the facial nerve and therefore should be considered during embolization of dural arteriovenous fistulae or tumors out of concern for facial paresis.

- The ascending pharyngeal artery may also form dangerous anastomoses with the ipsilateral vertebral artery. The meningeal branch is also responsible for vascular supply to the cranial nerve ganglia for the glossopharyngeal and vagus nerves; thus, caution should be exercised during embolization of this branch.

- The middle meningeal artery gives off a posteriorly directed petrosal branch at the level of the foramen spinosum, which travels along the middle fossa floor and can supply the geniculate ganglion. It is frequently a major contributor to the arterial supply of superior petrosal and transverse–sigmoid junction dural arteriovenous fistulae. Aberrant embolization may result in facial paresis. The main trunk of the middle meningeal artery courses anteriorly along the sphenoid wing toward the lateral calvarial dura and frequently anastomoses with the ophthalmic artery through the recurrent meningeal branch, which traverses the lateral aspect of the superior orbital fissure. Embolization of the middle meningeal artery may result in blindness through this dangerous collateral.

- The sphenopalatine segment can also give rise to branches to the ethmoidal sinus air cells. These branches frequently anastomose with anterior and posterior ethmoidal branches of the ophthalmic artery. Embolization with particulates during procedures for epistaxis or tumors may result in blindness or neurological sequelae through these dangerous collaterals.

# 3 Internal Carotid Artery

The internal carotid (IC) artery begins at the bifurcation of the common carotid artery at the same level in the neck as the origin of the external carotid artery. It lies first in the carotid triangle and medial to the anterior border of the sternocleidomastoid muscle and is covered by deep fascia. Proximally, the posterior belly of the digastric muscle and the stylohyoid muscle cross laterally over it. Distally, the IC artery lies medial to the styloglossus (or styloid process) and stylopharyngeus muscles, whereas the external carotid artery is positioned lateral to these muscles. At this point, the IC artery medially lies on the surface of the superior pharyngeal constrictor. At the base of the skull, the IC artery is more intimately related to the ninth cranial nerve, which passes over its lateral surface, and the inferior petrosal vein, whereas the internal jugular vein is more intimately related to the tenth and eleventh nerves.

The hypoglossal (XII) foramen is medial and slightly posterior to the entry of the IC artery to the cranial base. The IC artery and cranial nerves IX, X, XI, and XII are encased in a tough fibrous band at the base of the skull. The IC artery enters the petrous bone anterior and inferior to the cochlea and tympanum. It curves slightly upward and forward and then medial to pass under the gasserian ganglion coursing superiorly into the cavernous sinus. Usually, there is a thin osseous divider separating the gasserian ganglion from the IC canal. If the bony divider is deficient, a tough fibrous membrane connects the periosteum of the IC canal with the undersurface of the gasserian ganglion. This fibrous band is the carotid trigeminal ligament. At the base of the foramen lacerum, just prior to entry into the cavernous sinus, the IC artery, with its periosteum, is frequently attached firmly to the porous bone at the base of the foramen lacerum. This may account for dissections of the IC artery that originate in the neck or the base of the cranium terminating at the area of the foramen lacerum. In the carotid canal, at the cranial base, the IC artery has a larger diameter than the subsequent intradural distal portion of the IC. In the bony carotid canal, prior to entry into the cavernous sinus, the IC artery is sheathed in a tough periosteal membrane, within which are sympathetic nerves and venous sinuses. As the IC artery passes under the petrolingual ligament to enter the cavernous sinus, the periosteum of the IC flares like a trumpet to become continuous with the lining of the interior of the cavernous sinus.

The lateral portion of the periosteum of the IC bony canal lines the inner portion of the lateral wall of the cavernous sinus. The first division of the fifth cranial nerve and the third and fourth cranial nerves are embedded in this lateral wall. The sixth nerve is within the cavernous sinus and is attached to the IC by a very short, fine, fibrous ligament. The periosteum of the IC is also continuous with the dural floor of the sella turcica. The IC then passes just lateral and inferior to the pituitary fossa, grooving the body of the sphenoid bone, and then turning medial through the proximal ring and superiorly piercing the distal ring to enter the intradural space of the cranial vault. The cavernous sinus itself is separated from the medial pituitary body by a veil of dura descending from the roof to the floor of the cavernous sinus. It should be noted that the third and fourth cranial nerves travel through canals or dural sheaths in their course through the wall of the lateral cavernous sinus. The fourth nerve, as it passes out of the sheath of the wall of the cavernous sinus, goes superiorly and superficial to the annulus of Zinn to enter the orbit. The third nerve courses within the annulus of Zinn to bifurcate into a superior and inferior division within the apex of the orbit. Because the first division of the fifth nerve passes into the apex of the orbit, only the nasociliary division enters within the annulus of Zinn, whereas the remainder of the first division of the fifth nerve passes external to the annulus of Zinn to enter the orbital contents. The second division of the fifth nerve lies in a groove in the body of the sphenoid passing through the foramen rotundum into the inferior orbital fissure. Although the second division of the fifth nerve lies at the base of the lateral wall of the cavernous sinus, it is actually not part of the wall of the cavernous sinus.

There are smaller branches of the petrous portion of the IC artery, as well as the cavernous portion. They are difficult to find, even on injected specimens. The caroticotympanic branch is a small branch that pierces the tympanic cavity through a small foramen in the carotid canal. In addition, after a very short

vertical course in the cavernous sinus, the IC artery gives off the meningohypophyseal trunk. In the midportion of the horizontal IC artery in the cavernous sinus, the inferior lateral trunk arises superior and lateral to the sixth nerve in the cavernous sinus. It supplies the adjoining lateral dura and gasserian ganglion. There are small branches from the horizontal IC artery in the cavernous sinus passing to the floor of the sella turcica. There is an anterior meningeal branch to the dura of the lesser wing of the sphenoid.

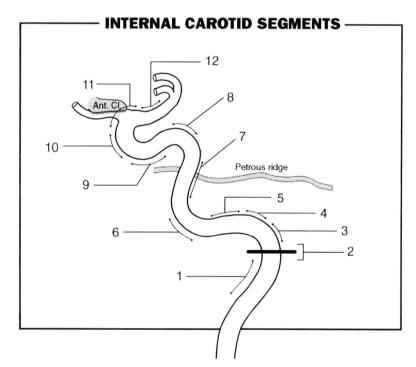

**INTERNAL CAROTID SEGMENTS**

**Fig. 3.1** Anatomical segments of the internal carotid artery.

1  cervical
2  skull entry zone
3  ascending petrous
4  genu petrous
5  pre-gasserian petrous
6  retro-gasserian petrous
7  lacerum
8  posterior cavernous genu
9  horizontal cavernous
10  anterior cavernous genu
11  carotid-ophthalmic triangle
12  supraclinoid

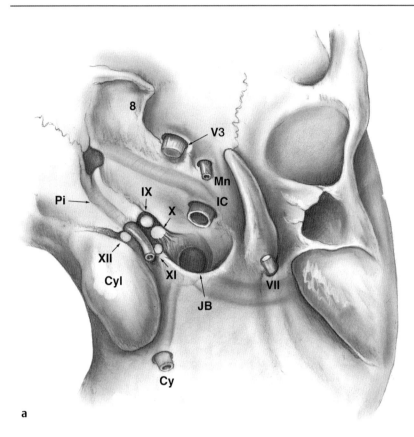

**Fig. 3.2** **(a)** View of the left side of the base of the cranium. Note inferior petrosal sinus (Pi) penetrating cranium in separate foramen, becoming the inferior petrosal vein in the neck, and eventually joining internal jugular vein.

Pi     inferior petrosal sinus
8      lateral pterygoid plate
V3     third division of fifth nerve
IX     ninth nerve
X      tenth nerve
XI     eleventh nerve
XII    twelfth nerve
JB     jugular bulb
Cyl    condyle
IC     internal carotid artery
Mn     middle meningeal artery
VII    seventh nerve
Cy     condyloid venous foramen

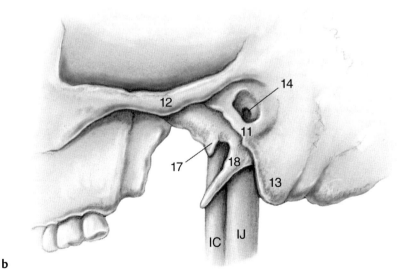

**Fig. 3.2** **(b)** A lateral view of the left cranial base showing the relationship of the styloid process to the internal carotid artery and the internal jugular vein. (Same as **Fig. 1.3b**.)

11     tympanic plate
12     zygomatic process
13     mastoid process
14     external auditory canal
17     crista tympanic
18     styloid process
IC     internal carotid artery
IJ     internal jugular vein

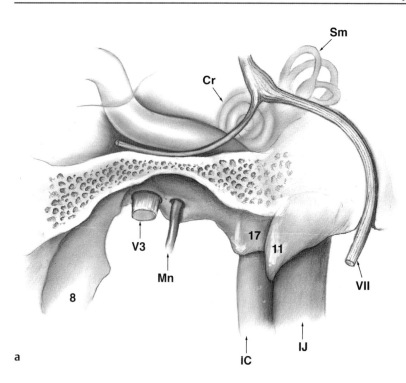

**Fig. 3.3 (a)** Left lateral view of the cranium. The basic relationships of the high cervical internal carotid artery, carotid artery entry zone, and initial petrous carotid are shown.

Cr   cochlea
IC   internal carotid artery
IJ   internal jugular vein
Mn  middle meningeal artery
Sm  semicircular canals
V3  third division of fifth nerve
8    lateral pterygoid plate
11   tympanic plate
17   crista tympanic
VII  seventh nerve

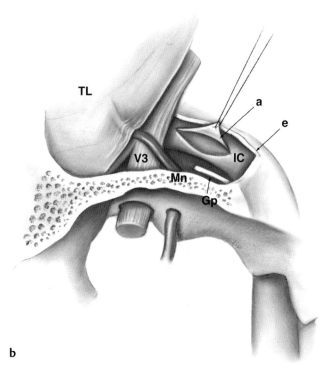

**Fig. 3.3 (b)** Left lateral view of the cranium.

a   cut periosteum of IC
e   bony window into carotid canal
V3  third division of fifth nerve
Gp  greater superficial petrosal nerve
IC  internal carotid artery
Mn  middle meningeal artery
TL  temporal lobe (dura)

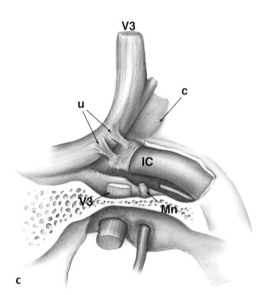

**Fig. 3.3   (c)** Left lateral view of the cranium.

IC   internal carotid artery
V3   third division of fifth nerve
Mn   middle meningeal artery
c   Meckel's cave (floor)
u   trigeminal carotid ligament

c

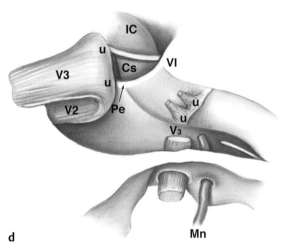

**Fig. 3.3   (d)** Left lateral view of the cranium.

Cs   cavernous sinus
IC   internal carotid artery
Pe   petro-lingual ligament
V2   second division of fifth nerve
V3   third division of fifth nerve
u   cut ends of trigeminal carotid ligament
VI   sixth nerve
Mn   middle meningeal artery

d

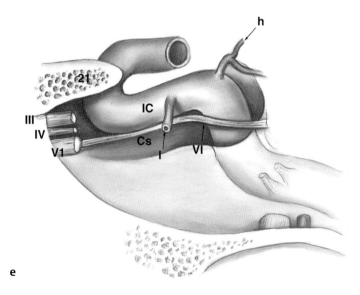

**Fig. 3.3   (e)** Left lateral view of the cranium.

Cs   cavernous sinus
IC   internal carotid artery
h   meningohypophyseal trunk
I   infero-lateral trunk
III   third nerve
IV   fourth nerve
V1   first division of fifth nerve
VI   sixth nerve
21   anterior clinoid

e

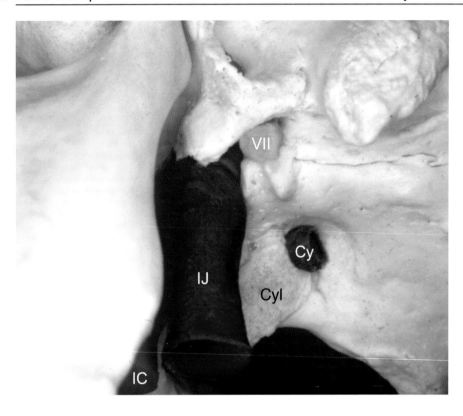

**Fig. 3.4** The internal carotid artery (IC) passes medial to the angle of the jaw, anterior to and medial to the internal jugular vein (IJ).

VII  seventh nerve exiting stylomastoid foramen
Cy  condyloid emissary vein
Cyl  condyle
IC  internal carotid artery
IJ  internal jugular vein

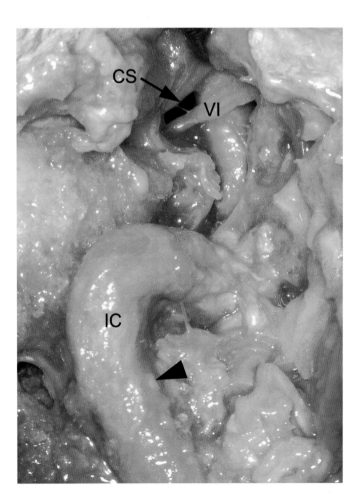

**Fig. 3.5** The right internal carotid artery (IC) with bone at the base of the skull removed, coursing superior and anterior into the cavernous sinus (CS).

VI  sixth nerve
Arrowhead  entry point into skull base

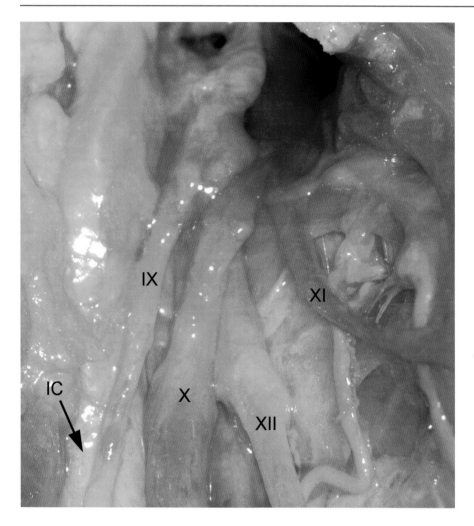

**Fig. 3.6** View of cranial nerves on left side exiting the jugular foramen medially with the internal jugular vein removed.

XI    eleventh nerve
X     tenth nerve
IX    ninth nerve; nerve IX courses over and lateral to internal carotid artery (IC); the hypoglossal nerve (XII) is seen descending deep to IX, X, XI and then to pass more superficial and over the external carotid artery (*not shown*)

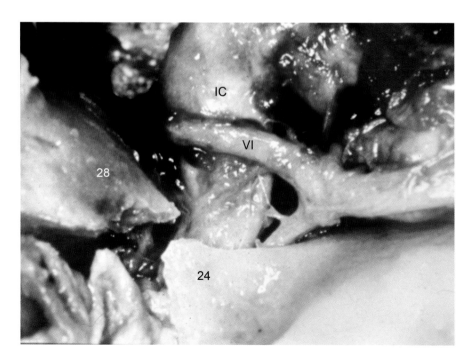

**Fig. 3.7** View of the internal carotid artery (IC) on the right as it passes the petrolingual region entering the cavernous sinus. All the dural membranes have been stripped away.

VI    sixth nerve
24    lingular process of the sphenoid bone
28    petrous apex

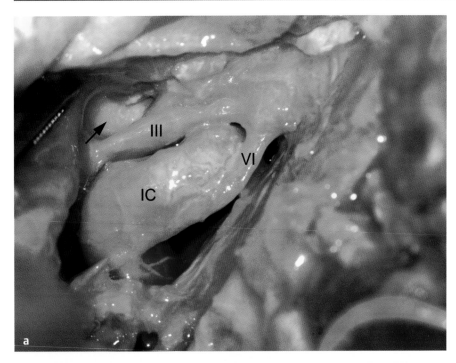

**Fig. 3.8** **(a)** Lateral view of the right internal carotid artery (IC) in the cavernous sinus and its intradural extension (*arrow*).

VI   sixth nerve
III  third nerve

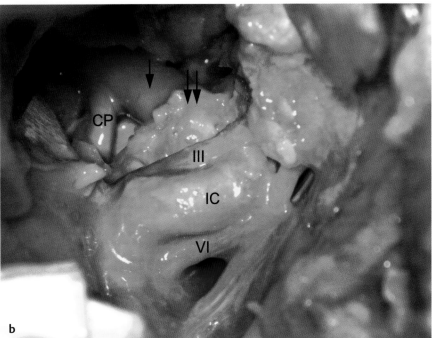

**Fig. 3.8** **(b)** The intracranial segment of the right internal carotid artery (*arrow*) just after exiting the distal dural ring (*double arrow*).

IC   cavernous internal carotid artery
CP   posterior communicating artery
III  third nerve
VI   sixth nerve

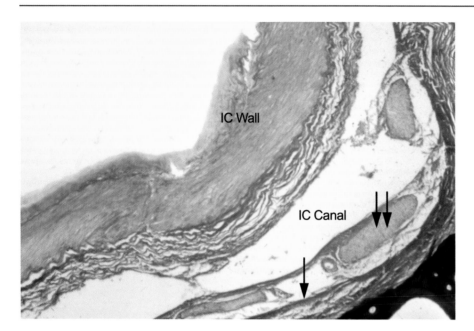

**Fig. 3.9** See **Fig. 3.18**. Photomicrograph of sagittal section of petrous internal carotid artery (IC). Arrow indicates the periosteum lining the internal carotid canal. Note the sympathetic plexus (*double arrows*) enveloped in the periosteal membranes.

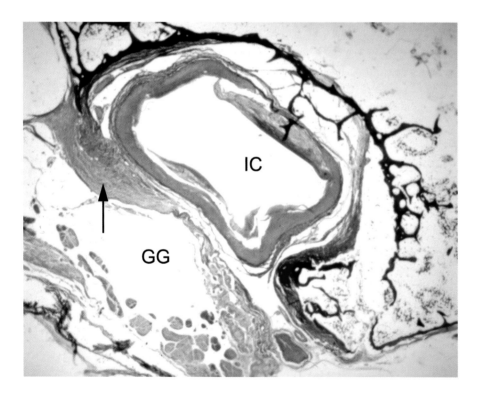

**Fig. 3.10** Cross section of internal carotid artery (IC) in bony canal with thick dural covering (*arrow*) separating it from the gasserian ganglion (GG).

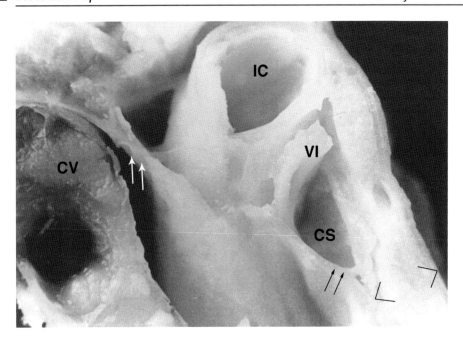

**Fig. 3.11** Coronal section through the clivus (CV) and posterior cavernous sinus (CS) as the internal carotid artery (IC) enters the posterior cavernous sinus. Note the flaring of the periosteum (*two sets of double arrows*) as the internal carotid artery enters the posterior cavernous sinus. The periosteum of the IC canal fuses with the medial portion of the lateral wall of the cavernous sinus (*opposing arrowheads*). Medially, the periosteum of the IC (*left double arrows*) is continuous with the dura of the medial posterior cavernous sinus.

VI  sixth nerve

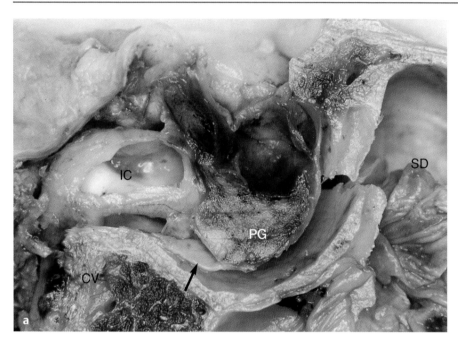

**Fig. 3.12** **(a)** Sagittal section looking medially at the left pituitary fossa. Arrow indicates the dura of the floor of the pituitary fossa that posteriorly and inferiorly is continuous with the periosteum of the internal carotid artery.

IC internal carotid artery
CV clivus
PG pituitary gland
SD sphenoid sinus

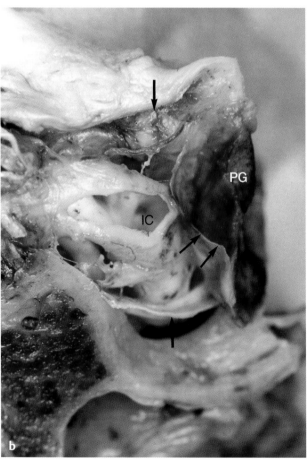

**Fig. 3.12** **(b)** Same specimen as **(a)**, but seen posteriorly. Double arrows indicate the dural veil that separates the pituitary gland from the internal carotid artery in the cavernous sinus, extending from the roof (*upper arrow*) to the floor (*lower arrow*) of the cavernous sinus.

IC internal carotid artery
PG pituitary gland

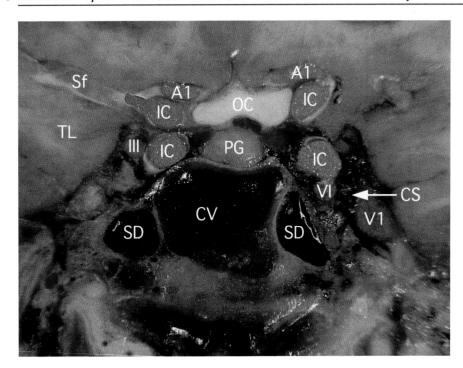

**Fig. 3.13** Coronal section through the cranial base at the level of the middle of the pituitary fossa and optic chiasm above.

A1   anterior cerebral artery
IC   internal carotid artery
OC   optic chiasm
CS   cavernous sinus
CV   clivus
PG   pituitary gland
SD   sphenoid sinus
Sf   Sylvian fissure
TL   temporal lobe
V1   first division of fifth nerve
VI   sixth nerve
III   third nerve

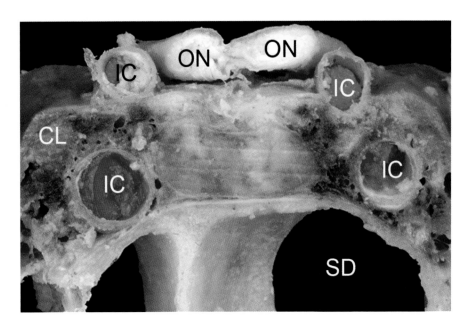

**Fig. 3.14** Coronal section through the cranial base at the level of sphenoid sinus (SD) and base of the anterior clinoid process (CL) viewed from posterior to anterior. Note that the diameter of the internal carotid artery (IC) decreases as it goes from the infraclinoid position to the supraclinoid position.

ON   optic nerve

## 3.1 Clinical Cases

### 3.1.1 Case 1

A middle-aged woman presented with increasing headaches and left-sided facial pain. Computed tomographic angiography (CTA) revealed a persistent trigeminal artery (PTA), and an angiogram confirmed the persistent trigeminal artery with an aneurysm in Meckel's cave. The aneurysm was embolized with coils, with resolution of her symptoms.

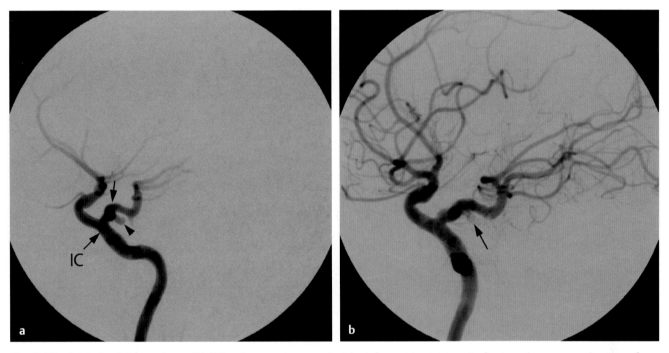

**Fig. 3.15** **(a)** Lateral internal carotid (IC) artery angiogram. Incidental persistent trigeminal artery (*upper arrow*) arising from the genu of the cavernous internal carotid artery (*lower arrow*). There is an aneurysm in the area of Meckel's cave (*arrowhead*). **(b)** Postembolization coiling of Meckel's cave aneurysm (*arrow*).

## 3.1.2 Case 2

A middle-aged woman presented with headaches, and magnetic resonance angiography (MRA) results suggestive of a paraclinoid aneurysm. The angiogram revealed a persistent otic artery supplying the anterior inferior cerebellar artery, as well as a small, irregular superior hypophyseal aneurysm. This was treated with flow diversion, resulting in resolution of her headaches.

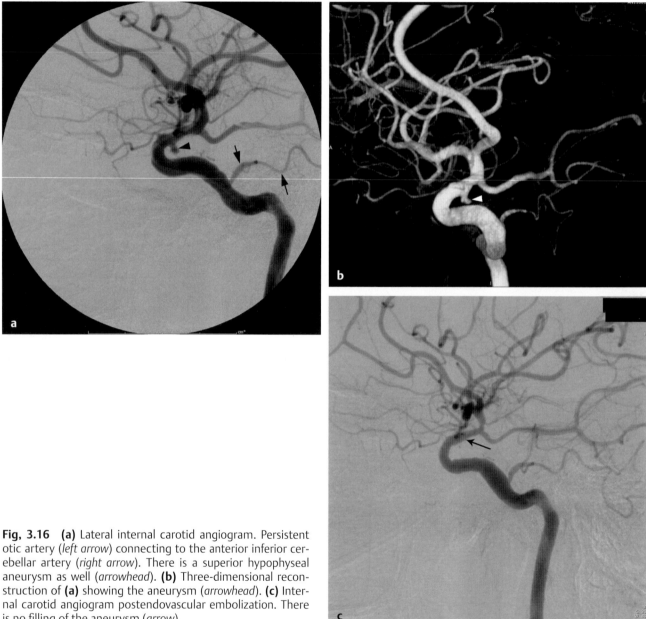

**Fig, 3.16** **(a)** Lateral internal carotid angiogram. Persistent otic artery (*left arrow*) connecting to the anterior inferior cerebellar artery (*right arrow*). There is a superior hypophyseal aneurysm as well (*arrowhead*). **(b)** Three-dimensional reconstruction of **(a)** showing the aneurysm (*arrowhead*). **(c)** Internal carotid angiogram postendovascular embolization. There is no filling of the aneurysm (*arrow*).

## 3.1.3 Case 3

A middle-aged woman presented with recurrent transient ischemic attacks with imbalance, visual symptoms, and numbness in the face and arm. Computed tomographic angiography revealed a persistent hypoglossal artery traversing the hypoglossal canal and supplying the entire posterior circulation.

Magnetic resonance imaging was negative for ischemic events. An angiogram confirmed high-grade stenosis of the persistent hypoglossal artery. This was treated through proximal protection and stent-assisted revascularization, with resolution of her presenting symptoms.

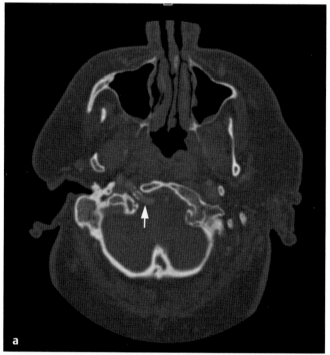

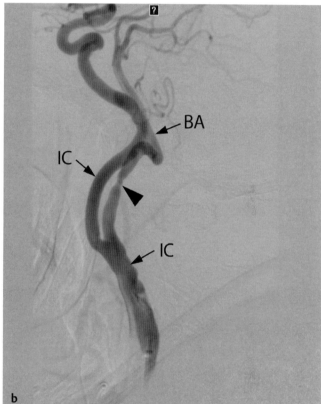

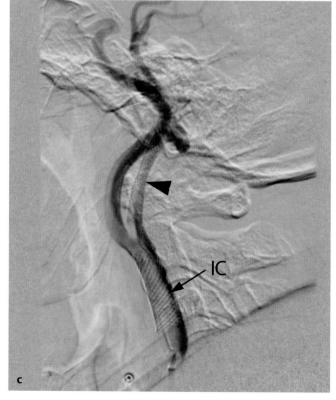

**Fig. 3.17** **(a)** Computed tomographic angiogram. A calcified, persistent right hypoglossal artery (*arrow*). **(b)** Digital subtraction carotid angiogram. The persistent hypoglossal artery (*arrowhead*) communicates with the basilar artery (BA) via the neck. Note stenosis of the hypoglossal artery (*arrowhead*). The internal carotid artery (IC) is also seen. **(c)** The IC artery and the persistent hypoglossal artery (*arrowhead*) are stented to eliminate the hypoglossal artery stenosis.

## 3.1.4 Case 4

A middle-aged man presented with an episode of amaurosis fugax. Computed tomographic angiography was concerning for pseudoocclusion. An angiogram confirmed complete occlusion of the cervical internal carotid (IC) artery with recanalization of the IC artery through collaterals from terminal branches of the ascending pharyngeal neuromeningeal trunk and the internal maxillary arteries. The patient was medically treated, resulting in resolution of symptoms and no hypoperfusion on vascular reserve testing.

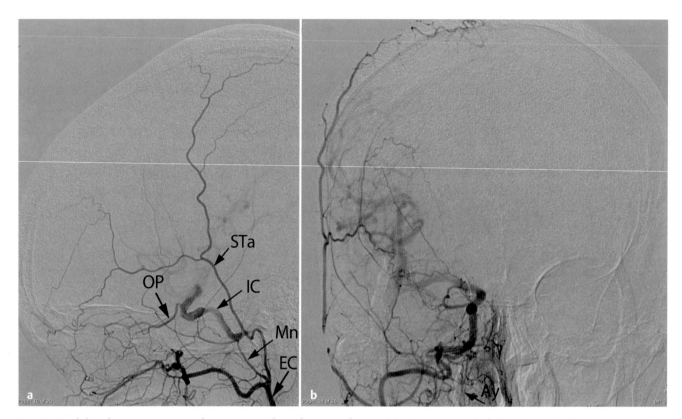

**Fig. 3.18** **(a)** Right common carotid angiogram. The right internal carotid (IC) artery is occluded in the neck. **(b)** Fine branches of the ascending pharyngeal artery (*arrow*) of the external carotid artery have collateral connections to the IC artery.

EC   external carotid artery
STa   superficial temporal artery
Mn   middle meningeal artery
OP   ophthalmic artery
Ay   ascending pharyngeal artery

## 3.1.5 Case 5

A middle-aged man presented with headaches and pulsatile tinnitis in the right ear. Magnetic resonance imaging (MRI) was concerning for increased vascularity around the right transverse sigmoid junction, with magnetic resonance venography suggesting occlusion of the right transverse sinus. An angiogram revealed an occlusion of the right transverse sinus with a dural arteriovenous fistula filled by branches from the meningohypophyseal trunk of the internal carotid artery and multiple external carotid artery branches, predominantly, the petrous branch of the middle meningeal artery (Mn) and posterior auricular and occipital arteries. Selective catheterization of the parietal Mn branch allowed direct arterial access to the blind venous fistulous pouch, which was embolized with a liquid embolic, resulting in obliteration of the fistula, including the superior petrosal sinus, with resolution of headaches and tinnitis.

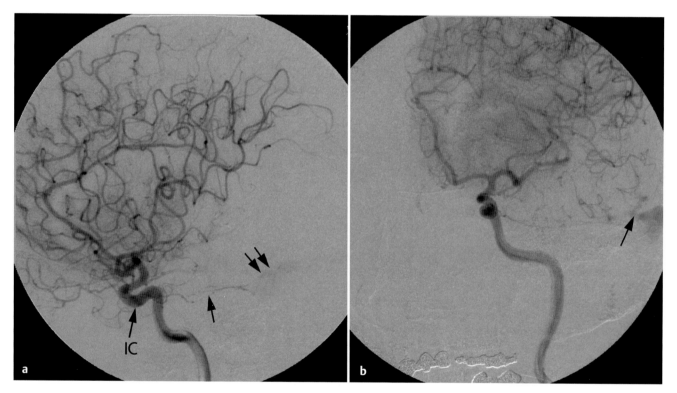

**Fig. 3.19** **(a)** Left lateral internal carotid angiogram. Arteriovenous fistula. The meningohypophyseal branch (*single arrow*) of the internal carotid (IC) artery drains as a fistula into the junction of the sigmoid and transverse sinus (*double arrows*). **(b)** Anteroposterior view of **(a)**. Note the arteriovenous junction of the fistula (*arrow*).

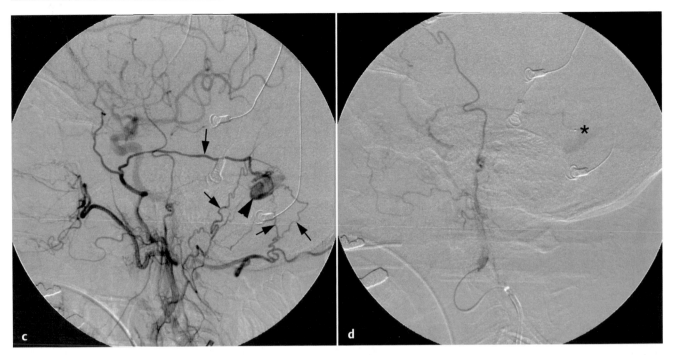

**Fig. 3.19** (*Continued*)   **(c)** Left selective external carotid angiogram showing the petrosal branch of the middle meningeal artery (*upper arrow*), the posterior auricular branch to the fistula, and transosseous branches of the occipital artery to the fistula (*right lower arrows*). The venous pouch of the fistula is seen (*arrowhead*). There are multiple arterial contributions (*arrows*) to the dural arteriovenous fistula. The transverse sigmoid junction (*arrowhead*) is also seen. **(d)** A microcatheter is seen at the fistula (*asterisk*).

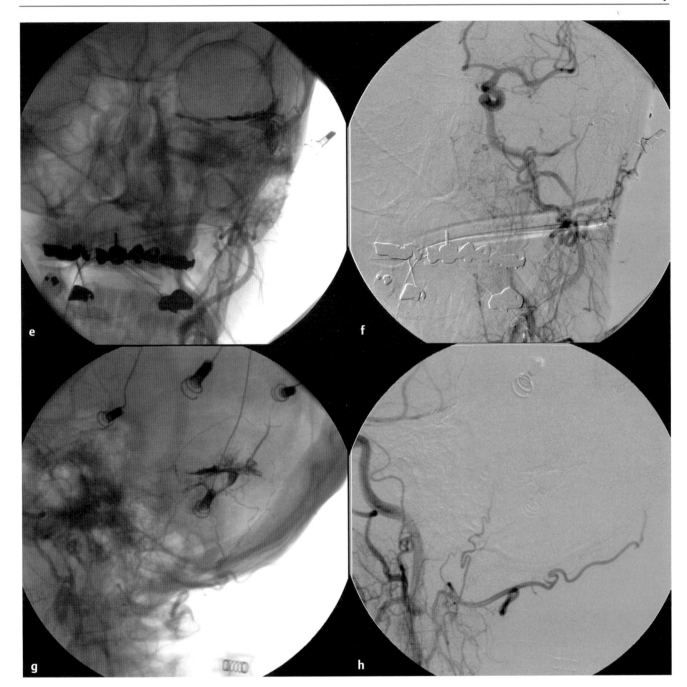

**Fig. 3.19** (*Continued*) **(e–h)** A right external carotid angiogram. A subtraction image of **(e)** shows no filling of the fistula.

## 3.1.6 Case 6

A young woman presented with presyncope and headaches. Magnetic resonance angiography revealed a large, petrous carotid artery aneurysm. This was treated with flow diversion, with resolution of her symptoms. Follow-up angiography revealed complete reconstruction of the native internal carotid artery.

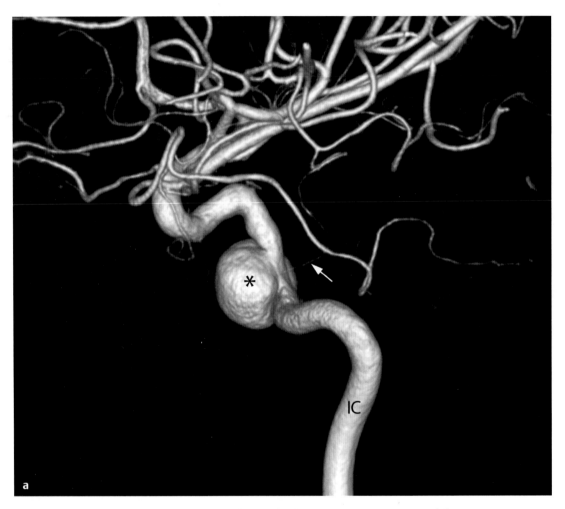

**Fig. 3.20** **(a)** Three-dimensional left internal carotid (IC) angiogram. A 10 × 14 mm left petrous IC artery aneurysm (*asterisk*) with anastomosis to the caroticotympanic branch (*arrow*).

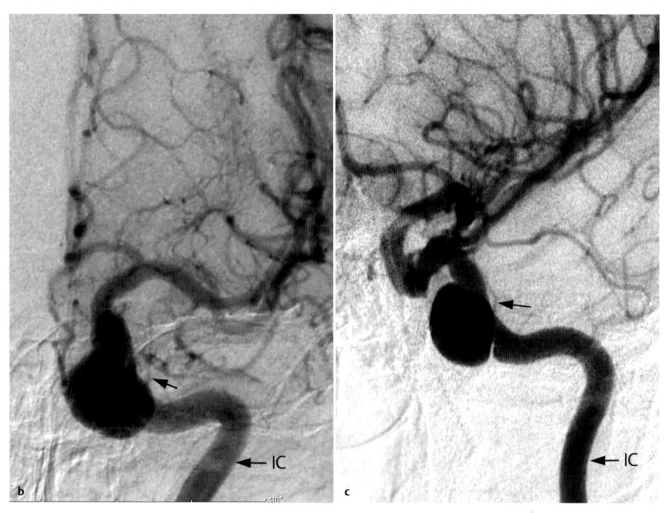

**Fig. 3.20** (*Continued*)   **(b)** Anteroposterior view of the left internal carotid (IC) artery angiogram. The caroticotympanic branch (*arrow*) is connected to the aneurysm. **(c)** Lateral view of **(b)**.

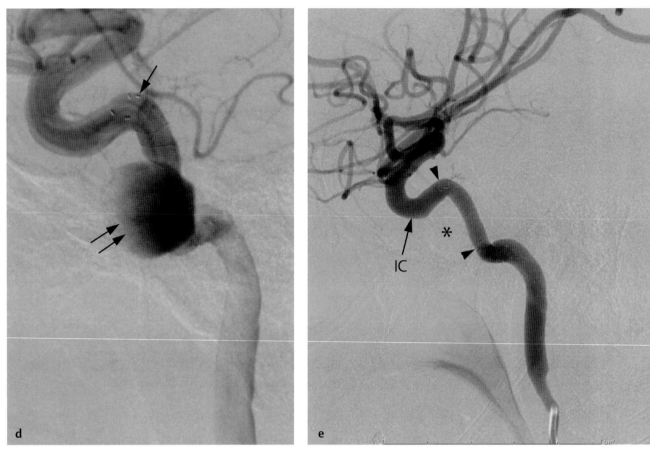

**Fig. 3.20** (*Continued*)    **(d)** A flow diverter (*upper arrow*) was placed across the aneurysm neck from the proximal cavernous internal carotid artery (IC) to the petrous portion. Immediate stasis was noted in the aneurysm (*double arrows*). **(e)** Follow-up left IC angiogram. Complete obliteration of the aneurysm (*asterisk*) and reconstruction of the IC artery. The flow diverter location is indicated (*arrowheads*).

## 3.1.7 Case 7

A young boy, while chasing his brother with a stick, fell, with the stick entering his mouth and posterior pharynx. Initially, he was neurologically intact, but by the time he presented to the emergency room he had developed left hemiplegia. Computed tomographic angiography demonstrated a right internal carotid (IC) artery dissection occlusion with secondary embolus occluding the right middle cerebral artery (MCA). He was immediately taken for endovascular recanalization. The IC artery was reconstituted with a cervical self-expanding stent, and the MCA thrombus was retrieved using a combination of stent retrieval and thromboaspiration. The patient made an excellent recovery with minimal hand weakness, which resolved by 3 months.

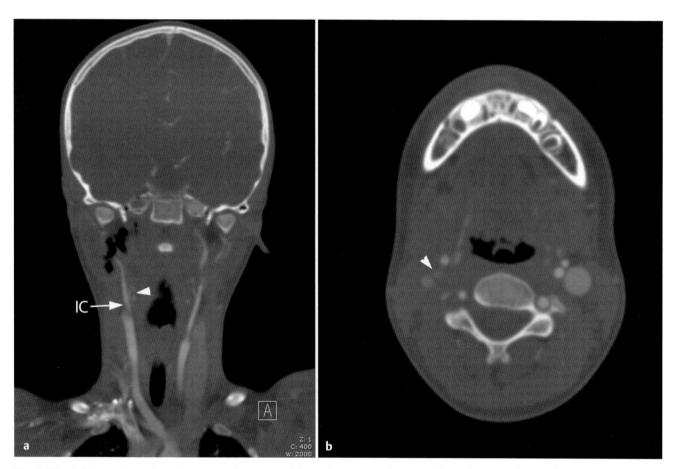

**Fig. 3.21** **(a)** Coronal section of computed tomographic angiogram. Occlusion of the right internal carotid (IC) artery with intimal flap (*arrowhead*). **(b)** Axial section. Arrowhead points to the intimal flap, a pseudoaneurysm resulting from direct injury to the internal carotid artery.

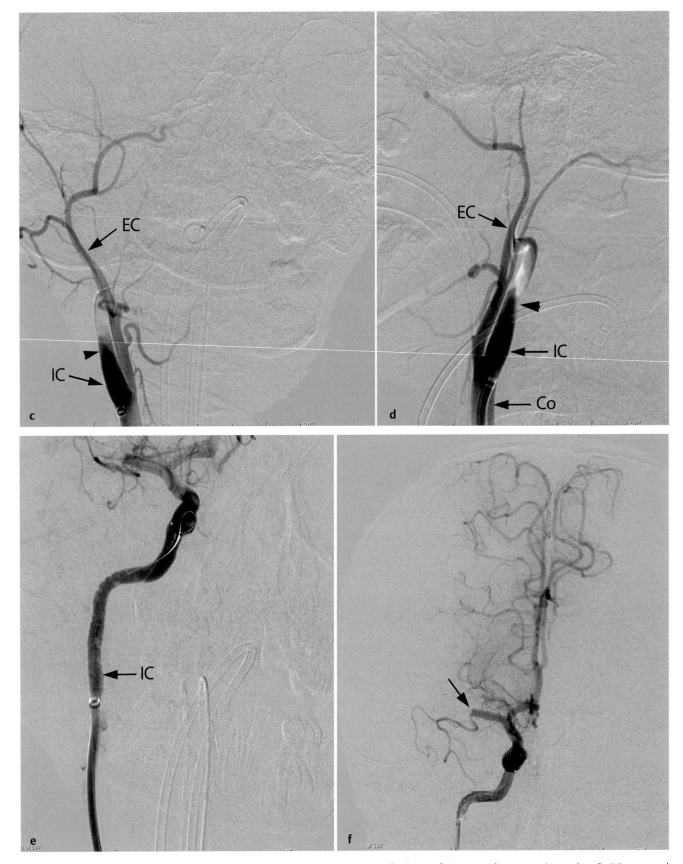

**Fig. 3.21** (*Continued*)   **(c)** Right common carotid (Co) angiogram. Proximal extent of IC artery dissection (*arrowhead*). EC, external carotid artery. **(d)** Lateral view. **(e)** Self-expanding stent inserted into the right IC artery. **(f)** A right middle cerebral artery embolic occlusion (*arrow*) is now evident.

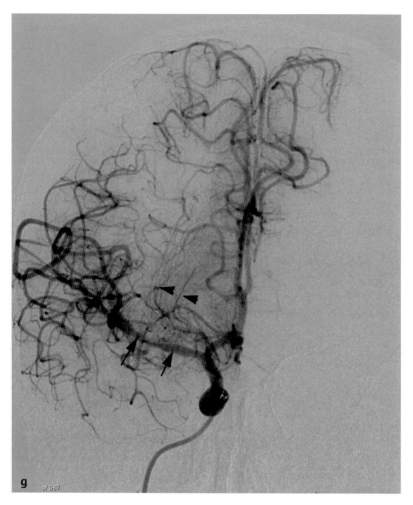

**Fig. 3.21** (*Continued*)   **(g)** The right middle cerebral artery M1 segment (*lower arrows*) is reconstituted with a microcatheter self-expanding stent retriever. The lenticulostriate arteries (*double arrowheads*) are filling.

## Clinical Pearls

- The uncommon persistent fetal connection between the carotid and posterior circulation that is most caudally located is the persistent proatlantal artery, which connects the cervical internal carotid (IC) artery to the vertebral artery, typically over the C1 lamina.

  The uncommon persistent fetal connection between the carotid and posterior circulation that is next cranially located is the persistent hypoglossal artery, which connects the terminal cervical IC artery to the vertebral artery through the hypoglossal canal.

- Tumors of the carotid body, typically glomus tumors and schwannomas of the sympathetic chain and ninth and tenth nerves, develop in the space between the external and internal carotid arteries, splaying these two vessels.

  The IC artery enters the petrous bone anterior and inferior to the cochlea and tympanum. There is a sharp bend from the vertically oriented cervical carotid to the horizontal and medially directed petrous IC artery in the proximal petrous canal

- The most common location of arterial dissections is the junction of the mobile cervical and adherent petrous segments of the IC artery. During endovascular repair of dissections in this region, the key dissection initiation site coverage by stents is hampered because carotid artery stents cannot be delivered around this bend; many times, additional stent types are required to navigate this bend.

  A rarely seen IC branch called the vidian artery pierces the foramen lacerum to travel along the greater superficial petrosal nerve through the vidian canal to the sphenopalatine ganglion.

- This ligament may account for dissections of the IC artery that originate in the neck or the base of the cranium terminating at the area of the foramen lacerum. The vidian artery may be enlarged in the dural arteriovenous fistulae and proximal IC artery occlusions, providing collateral flow from the internal maxillary artery. This artery may also serve as a possible dangerous anastomosis during embolization of internal maxillary artery branches for head and neck tumors and epistaxis.

  The greater and lesser petrosal nerves that carry preganglionic fibers from the seventh and ninth cranial nerves lie alongside the terminal horizontal petrous IC artery underneath the gasserian ganglion, and immediately below them is the eustachian tube, which travels deep and parallel to these structures.

- The horizontal segment of the petrous IC artery is frequently poorly covered by a bony roof and may be exposed and injured during subtemporal petrous extradural dissection, such as during a middle fossa approach for Meckel's cave or acoustic tumors, or during a Kawase approach for clival lesions. This segment of the IC artery has also been used for an IC-to-IC bypass using interposition grafts.

- Aneurysms of the cavernous carotid artery will frequently present with compressive symptoms of the cranial nerves within the cavernous sinus or its wall, the sixth cranial nerve being the most common nerve affected.

- The caroticotympanic branch is enlarged in cases of glomus tympanicum, dural arteriovenous fistulae, or cervical IC artery occlusions filling the IC through collaterals from neuromeningeal branches of the ascending pharyngeal and labrynthine branches of the anterior inferior cerebellar artery.

  In addition, after a very short vertical course in the cavernous sinus, the IC artery gives off the meningohypophyseal trunk. This trunk rapidly divides into the inferior hypophyseal artery, the tentorial branch of Bernasconi and Cassinari, and clival branches, which travel along the superior and inferior petrosal trunks. The clival and tentorial branches have rich anastomoses with terminal branches of the ascending pharyngeal (neuromeningeal trunk) artery, as well as meningeal branches of the occipital and vertebral arteries. The most cranial fetal IC–VB anastomosis, which typically regresses, is the persistent trigeminal artery, which arises just proximal to the menigohypophyseal trunk and travels through Meckel's cave into the posterior fossa.

- The inferior hypophyseal artery can be thrombosed during pregnancy, resulting in pituitary apoplexy (Sheehan's syndrome). In addition, the tentorial branches (of Bernasconi and Cassinari) are enlarged in tentorial arteriovenous fistulae and tentorial meningiomas. Embolization of this branch is very difficult due to the severe tortuosity of the proximal trunk, and is dangerous given the risks of reflux into the cavernous internal carotid artery and neurological injury through inadvertant embolization through collaterals of cranial nerve ganglia.

- The inferolateral trunk anastomoses with terminal branches of the internal maxillary artery through branches traveling through the foramen rotundum and the superior orbital fissure. These can be hypertrophied during indirect cavernous arteriovenous fistulae or meningeal tumors. This artery also plays a vital role, providing collaterals to a cavernous IC artery in cases of proximal cervical IC artery occlusion.

# 4 Carotid–Ophthalmic Triangle

The carotid–ophthalmic triangle is defined as the space through which courses the ophthalmic artery from the internal carotid artery to the optic strut. The roof of the triangle is the optic nerve, the medial wall is the body of the sphenoid bone, the lateral wall is the proximal anterior clinoid process, and the floor of the triangle is the internal carotid artery along with the distal dural ring. Just below and within this space, the internal carotid artery changes its orientation from posterior medially directed flow to posterior laterally directed flow. This dramatic change in orientation is pertinent to understanding the detailed local anatomy, as well as the change in flow direction. The course of the internal carotid artery in the carotid–ophthalmic triangle grooves the body of the sphenoid bone and is in close proximity to the sphenoid sinus as well.

## 4.1 Ophthalmic Artery

The ophthalmic artery usually arises in the subdural space from the medial and superior surface of the internal carotid artery just as the internal carotid artery emerges from the distal ring. This also positions the ophthalmic artery, at its origin, inferior and medial to the optic nerve. However, other variations of the origin of the ophthalmic artery include: (1) lateral to the optic nerve, (2) partial epidural and subdural, (3) totally below the distal ring in the epidural space, or (4) from the cavernous internal carotid artery. In the latter case, the artery enters the orbit through a separate bony canal. Although rare, the ophthalmic artery may be absent, or the total blood supply in the ophthalmic distribution may be via branches from the middle meningeal artery.

At the origin of the ophthalmic artery, there is an initial short vertical limb followed by a longer horizontal limb running intradurally for approximately 4 mm. In the most common configuration, the ophthalmic artery initially is inferior-medial to the optic nerve and moves laterally as it courses anteriorly through the optic foramen (leaving the carotid–ophthalmic triangle), piercing the dura and entering the orbit.

In the orbit, the ophthalmic artery turns superior to the optic nerve to the medial wall of the orbit. The anterior and posterior ethmoidal arteries arise from the ophthalmic artery along the medial border of the orbit. The anterior ethmoidal artery most commonly arises from the artery that is destined to become the supratrochlear artery. It may arise less frequently from the supraorbital artery. The anterior ethmoidal artery enters the anterior ethmoidal foramen into the ethmoid sinus with an invagination of the periorbita. Upon entering the foramen, the anterior ethmoidal artery courses along the roof of the anterior ethmoidal sinus, supplying the mucosa. The anterior ethmoidal artery continues on to supply the anterior fossa dura and then curves inferiorly along the medial aspect of the ethmoidal sinuses to supply the nasal mucosa. The anterior ethmoidal artery may contribute to the mucosa of the frontal sinus.

The posterior ethmoidal artery is smaller in caliber but greater in length than the anterior ethmoidal artery. Typically, the posterior ethmoidal artery arises directly from the intraorbital ophthalmic artery, but it may arise from the supratrochlear artery or be absent. The posterior ethmoidal artery also enters its foramen with an invagination of the periorbita. After entering the foramen to the posterior ethmoid sinus, the posterior ethmoidal artery courses along the roof of the ethmoid sinus and supplies the mucosa. It may supply the anterior fossa dura or nasal mucosa.

## 4.2 Superior Hypophyseal Artery

Within the carotid–ophthalmic triangle, the superior hypophyseal artery, consisting of one to three small vessels, originates from the medial aspect of the internal carotid artery 4 to 5 mm after the origin of the ophthalmic artery. The superior hypophyseal artery supplies the pituitary stalk. In addition, it can give small branches to the optic chiasm and optic nerve.

The optic nerve itself has a visor-like ligament (the falciform ligament) attached to the superior edge of the optic foramen. It may measure up to 4 mm at its widest point, and its resection exposes more of the superior surface of the intradural optic nerve.

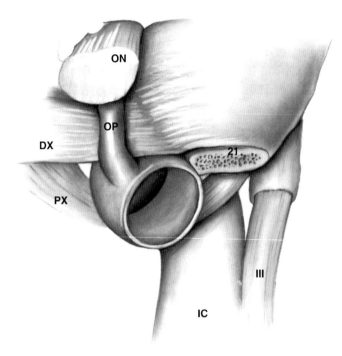

**Fig. 4.1** Superior view of the right internal carotid (IC) artery with the roof of the cavernous sinus dura removed. Part of the anterior clinoid tip has been removed.

III  third nerve
21  anterior clinoid
DX  distal ring
ON  optic nerve
OP  ophthalmic artery
PX  proximal ring

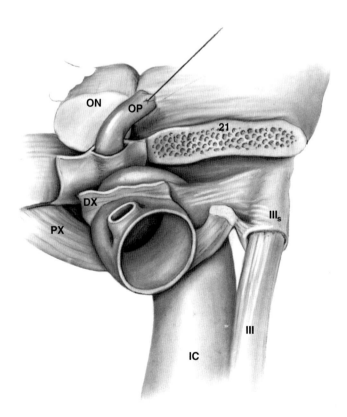

**Fig. 4.2** Superior view of the internal carotid artery with more extensive removal of the anterior clinoid exposing the relationship of the third nerve sheath to the proximal ring. A thin veil of dura extends from the third nerve sheath to the lateral internal carotid artery. Also note the attachment of the third nerve sheath to the proximal ring.

III  third nerve
III$_s$  third nerve sheath
21  anterior clinoid
DX  distal ring
ON  optic nerve
OP  ophthalmic artery
PX  proximal ring
IC  internal carotid artery

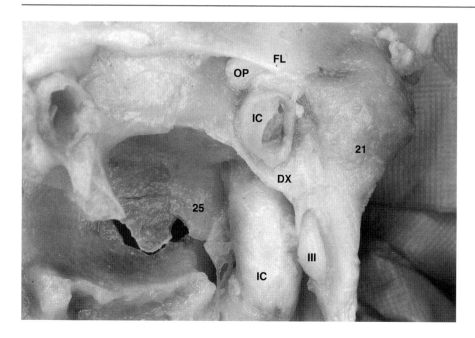

**Fig. 4.3** Superior view of the right parasellar internal carotid artery coursing through the cavernous sinus, piercing the distal ring, and entering the carotid–ophthalmic triangle. The pituitary gland has been removed from the pituitary fossa and the roof of the cavernous sinus over the parasellar internal carotid artery has been removed.

25  pituitary fossa
21  anterior clinoid
III  third nerve
DX  distal ring
FL  falciform ligament
IC  internal carotid artery
OP  optic nerve

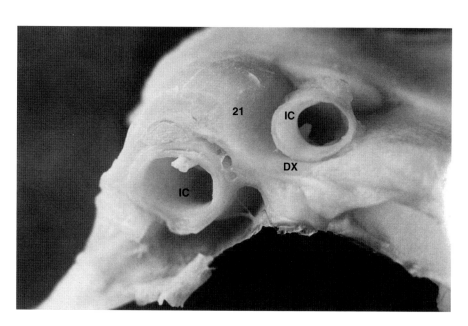

**Fig. 4.4** A cross section of the internal carotid artery as it appears below the anterior clinoid and then in the supraclinoid portion medial to the anterior clinoid process. Note the decrease in diameter of the internal carotid artery from its infraclinoid portion to its paraclinoid portion in the carotid–ophthalmic triangle.

21  anterior clinoid
DX  distal ring
IC  internal carotid artery

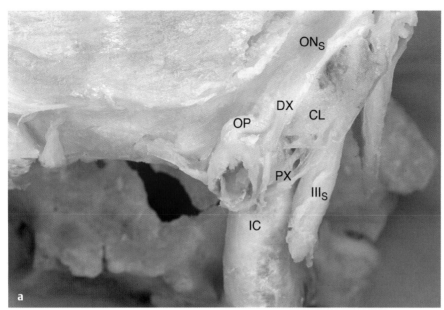

**Fig. 4.5** **(a)** Superior lateral view of the right carotid–ophthalmic triangle with a portion of the anterior clinoid removed, exposing the relationship between the distal ring and the proximal dural ring and the internal carotid artery. The optic nerve has been removed, and the ophthalmic artery can be seen penetrating the dural sheath as it courses medial to lateral.

III$_s$  third nerve sheath
DX  distal ring
IC  internal carotid artery
ON$_s$  optic nerve sheath
OP  ophthalmic artery
PX  proximal ring
CL  anterior clinoid

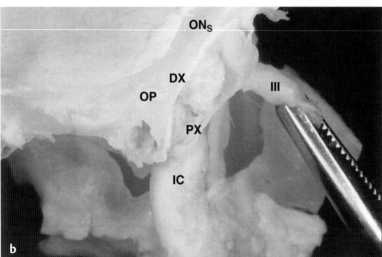

**Fig. 4.5** **(b)** The third nerve sheath has been partially resected, and the attachment of the proximal dural ring to the sheath of the third nerve is shown.

III  third nerve
DX  distal ring
IC  internal carotid artery
ON$_s$  optic nerve sheath
OP  ophthalmic artery
PX  proximal ring

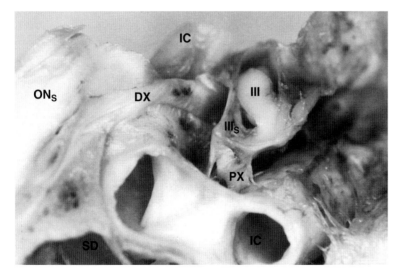

**Fig. 4.6** Inferior view of the right internal carotid artery as it courses through the anterior cavernous sinus piercing the distal dural ring and entering the subdural space above. Note again the attachment of the third nerve sheath to the proximal dural ring.

III  third nerve
III$_s$  third nerve sheath
DX  distal ring
IC  internal carotid artery
ON$_s$  optic nerve sheath
PX  proximal ring
SD  sphenoid sinus

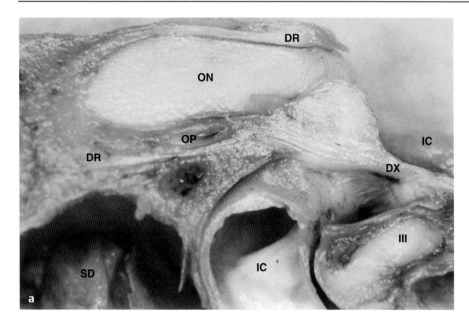

**Fig. 4.7** **(a)** A photo of a sagittal section through the region of the optic strut as the internal carotid artery courses superiorly through the distal dural ring. Lateral view of left side.

III   third nerve
DR   dura
DX   distal ring
IC   internal carotid artery
ON   optic nerve
OP   ophthalmic artery
SD   sphenoid sinus

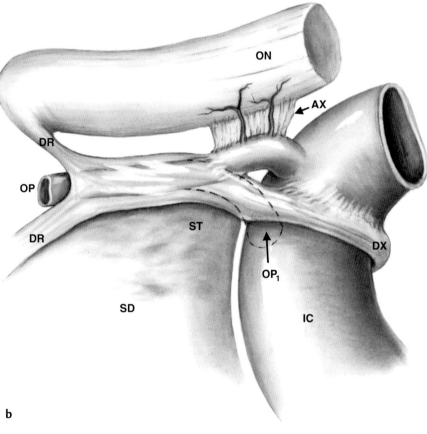

**Fig. 4.7** **(b)** An illustration similar to the photo in **(a)** showing the internal carotid artery piercing the distal dural ring and the relationship of the surrounding structures in the carotid–ophthalmic triangle of the left internal carotid artery (lateral view).

AX   arachnoid
DR   dura
DX   distal ring
IC   internal carotid artery
ON   optic nerve
OP   ophthalmic artery
OP$_1$   alternate origin of ophthalmic artery
SD   sphenoid sinus
ST   optic strut

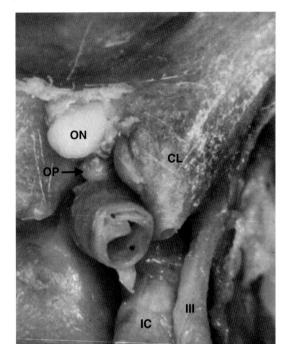

**Fig. 4.8** **(a)** A superior view of the right internal carotid artery as it goes from infraclinoid to paraclinoid in the carotid–ophthalmic triangle.

OP  ophthalmic artery
III  third nerve
CL  anterior clinoid
IC  internal carotid artery
ON  optic nerve

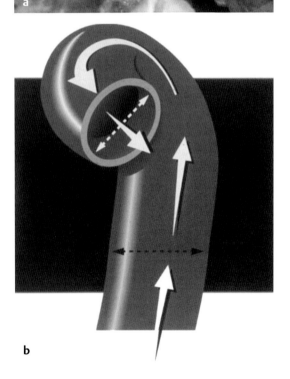

**Fig. 4.8** **(b)** A graphic representation of the change in flow direction and diameter as the artery goes from infraclinoid to paraclinoid and supraclinoid.

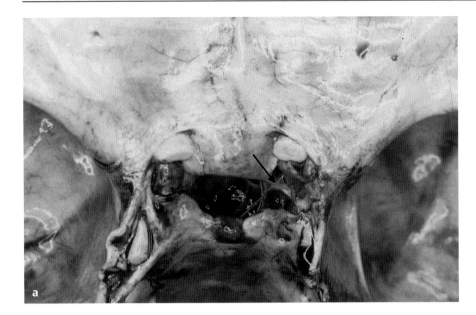

**Fig. 4.9** **(a)** Necropsy photo of the region of the sella turcica showing the superior hypophyseal artery (*arrow*) on the right going medially and posteriorly to enter the pituitary stalk.

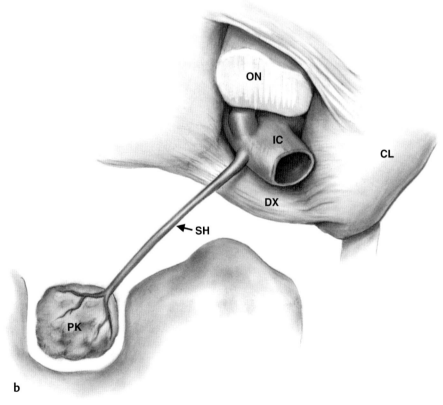

**Fig. 4.9** **(b)** Drawing of necropsy photo **(a)** showing course of superior hypophyseal artery.

CL   anterior clinoid
DX   distal ring
IC   internal carotid artery
ON   optic nerve
PK   pituitary stalk
SH   superior hypophyseal artery

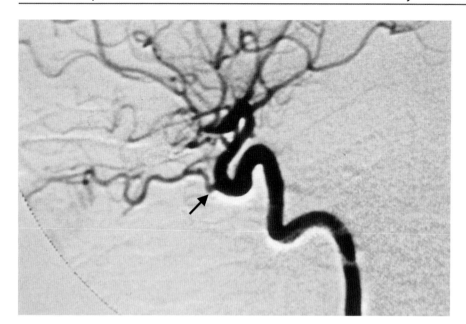

**Fig. 4.10** Right internal carotid artery angiogram showing an intracavernous origin of the ophthalmic artery (*arrow*).

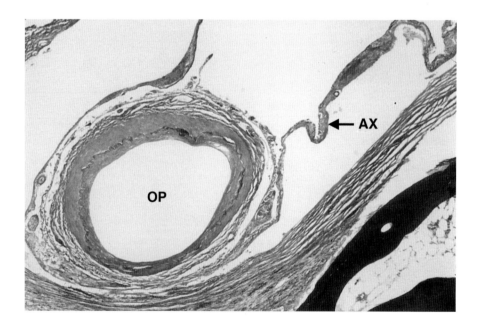

**Fig. 4.11** A photomicrograph of a cross section of the ophthalmic artery (OP) as it lies in the carotid–ophthalmic triangle with its arachnoid veil (AX) extending superiorly.

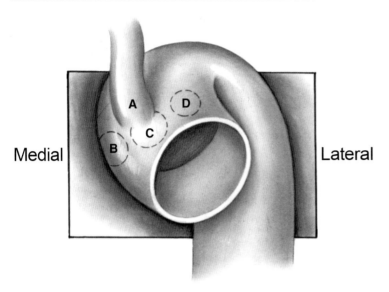

**Fig. 4.12** Variations in the origin of the ophthalmic artery as it might arise in the carotid–ophthalmic triangle (right side).

A  common
B  occasional
C  common
D  rare

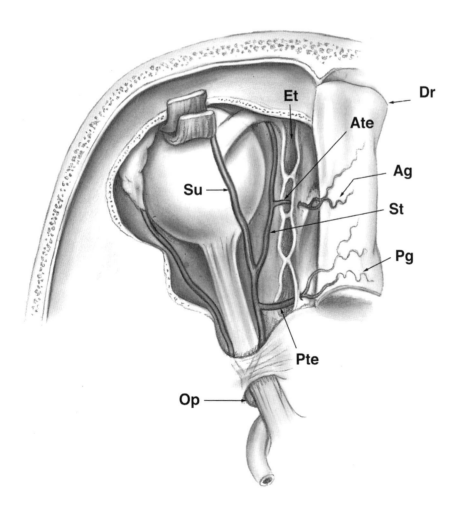

**Fig. 4.13** Superior view of the left orbit. Note the anterior meningeal (Ag) and posterior meningeal (Pg) branches of the ethmoidal arteries.

Ate  anterior ethmoidal artery
Dr  dura
Et  ethmoid sinus
Op  ophthalmic artery
Pte  posterior ethmoidal artery
St  supratrochlear artery
Su  supraorbital artery

## 4.3 Clinical Cases

### 4.3.1 Case 1

A middle-aged woman was found to have a transient ischemic attack affecting her right hemisphere with left-sided weakness and numbness, which resolved. The workup, including magnetic resonance angiography, revealed a giant paraclinoid aneurysm. The angiogram revealed a multicompartmental aneurysm affecting the entire paraclinoidal segment with aneurysmal outpouchings in the cavernous, clinoidal, and supraclinoidal segments. The patient was treated through flow diversion with three overlapping devices with immediate flow stasis in all separate compartments of the aneurysm. Delayed angiography revealed complete obliteration of all compartments and reconstruction of the internal carotid artery. The patient remained neurologically stable without recurrent problems or residual deficits.

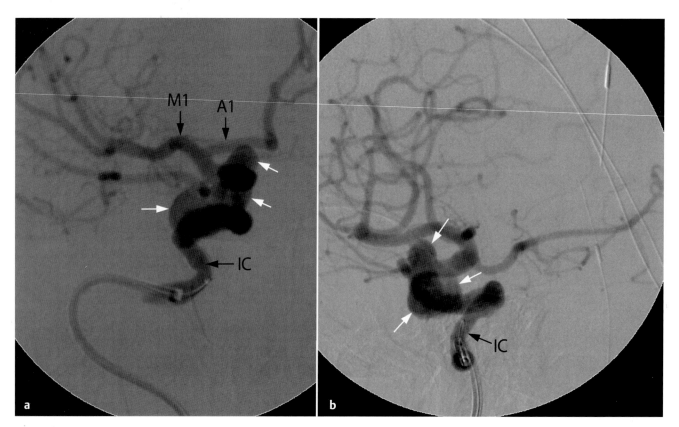

**Fig. 4.14** **(a)** Anteroposterior view of a right internal carotid angiogram with a guidewire in a giant internal carotid aneurysm (*arrows*) with outpouches into the distal cavernous sinus, internal carotid clinoidal segment, and supraclinoidal segment. IC, internal carotid artery; M1, middle cerebral artery; A1, anterior cerebral artery. **(b)** Lateral view of **(a)**.

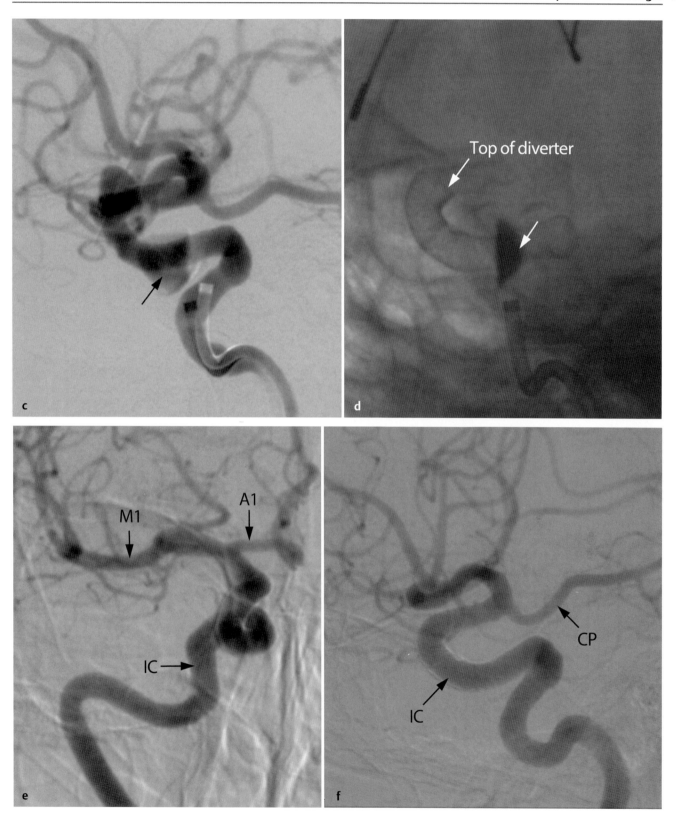

**Fig. 4.14** (*Continued*)   **(c)** Three overlapping flow diverters deployed into the right internal carotid artery. Immediate contrast stasis in the aneurysm (*arrow*) occurred. **(d)** Intraprocedural delayed fluoroscopic image demonstrates a "half-moon" sign in the aneurysm (*arrow*). **(e)** Delayed anteroposterior view of the right internal carotid (IC) angiogram in the same procedure as in **(d)**. Complete obliteration of the aneurysm. A1, anterior cerebral artery; M1, middle cerebral artery. **(f)** Lateral view of **(e)**. CP, right posterior communicating artery.

## 4.3.2 Case 2

A young woman was found to have a superior hypophyseal aneurysm during screening after her mother died of a ruptured intracranial aneurysm. The aneurysm was confirmed by angiography and then treated through stent-assisted coil embolization. Delayed angiography revealed complete obliteration of the aneurysm. The patient remained asymptomatic.

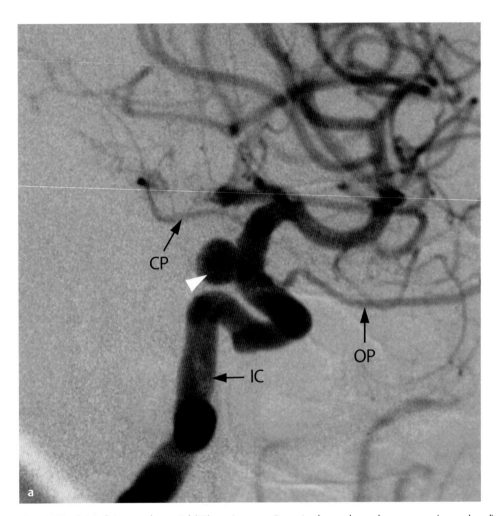

**Fig. 4.15** **(a)** Left internal carotid (IC) angiogram. Superior hypophyseal aneursym (*arrowhead*).

OP   ophthalmic artery
CP   left posterior communicating artery

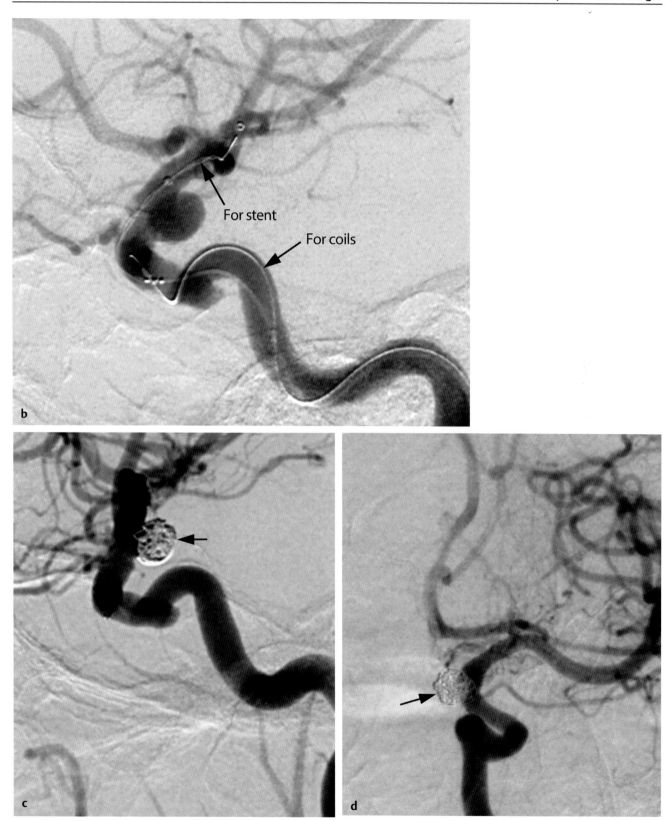

**Fig. 4.15** (*Continued*)   **(b)** Two microcatheters (*arrows*) in the left internal carotid artery. One is for deployment of the stent, and the other is for the coils. **(c)** Lateral view of the left internal carotid angiogram. Successful coiling of the aneurysm (*arrow*). **(d)** Anteroposterior view of **(c)**.

### 4.3.3 Case 3

A woman presented with increasing headaches and eye pressure. Magnetic resonance imaging revealed a large anterior cranial fossa venous varix draining into the superior sagittal sinus. Angiography revealed an anterior cranial fossa dural arteriovenous fistula fed by both ophthalmic arteries through their ethmoidal branches, with retrograde intracranial venous flow and a large venous varix. The patient underwent a craniotomy for clip ligation of the fistula with resul-

tant cure and resolution of symptoms. Although rare, the ophthalmic artery may be absent, or the total blood supply in the ophthalmic distribution may be via a recurrent meningeal branch arising from the middle meningeal artery in the superior orbital fissure. A rare variant of the ophthalmic artery, aberrantly called the dorsal ophthalmic artery, may arise entirely from the cavernous carotid artery and is a developmental remnant of the maxillary artery.

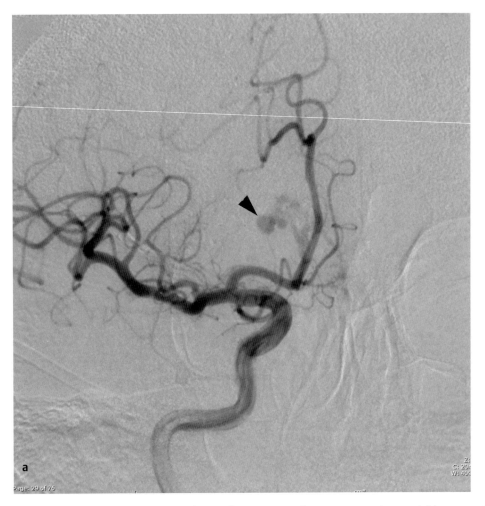

**Fig. 4.16** **(a)** Oblique right internal carotid angiogram. There is an anterior cranial base arteriovenous fistula with a venous varix (*arrowhead*).

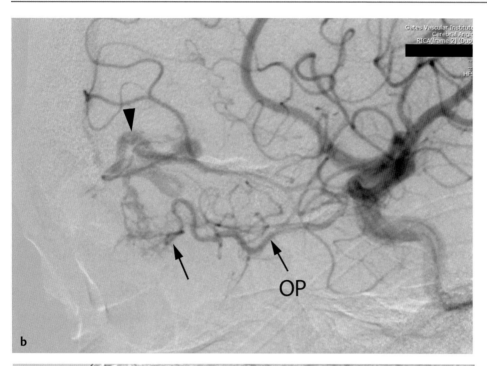

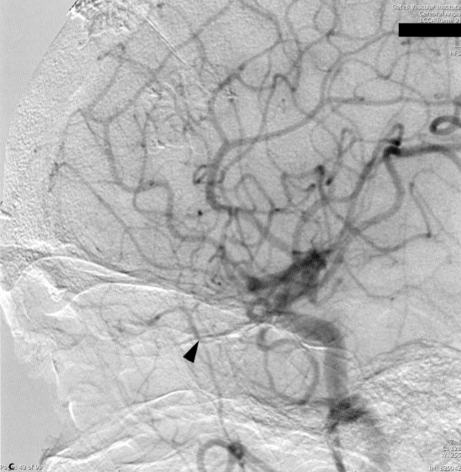

**Fig. 4.16** (*Continued*)   **(b)** Lateral view of **(a)**. The anterior ethmoidal branches (*arrow*) of the ophthalmic artery (OP) are supplying the dural arteriovenous fistula. Venous varix (*arrowhead*). **(c)** Postcraniotomy for the arteriovenous dural fistula. Reduction in size of the ophthalmic artery (*arrowhead*). Fistula does not fill.

## Clinical Pearls

- The anterior and posterior ethmoidal arteries extensively anastomose with the terminal ethmoidal branches of the internal maxillary artery and form dangerous collaterals to be identified prior to embolization for head and neck tumors and for epistaxis. In addition, these vessels are frequently involved in dural arteriovenous fistulas of the anterior cranial fossa, and, because of the risk to the retinal branches, are best treated through craniotomy and ligation of venous outflow. The ophthalmic artery is a key collateral that supplies intracranial in cases of proximal occlusion. By the same token, occlusion of the ophthalmic artery during flow diversion of paraclinoid aneurysms rarely results in retinal ischemic events because of extensive collaterals from the external carotid artery.

- Superior hypophyseal artery aneurysms are differentiated from ophthalmic artery aneurysms by their orientation. Hypophyseal aneurysms are directed medioinferiorly, whereas ophthalmic aneurysms are directed superolaterally. Therefore, ophthalmic artery aneurysms are more likely to cause compression of the ipsilateral optic nerve, whereas large hypophyseal aneurysms may compress the contralateral optic nerve. During craniotomy for clipping, ophthalmic aneurysms may be best approached from the ipsilateral direction, whereas smaller hypophyseal aneurysms are best seen from a contralateral approach.

# 5 Posterior Communicating Artery and Anterior Choroidal Artery

## 5.1 Posterior Communicating Artery

The posterior communicating artery (CP) typically originates from the inferior lateral wall of the internal carotid artery, just a few millimeters distal to the tip of the anterior clinoid process and as the internal carotid artery emerges under the optic nerve. However, the CP origin may be more proximal and hidden under the anterior clinoid process. The CP itself may course laterally, adjacent to the third nerve, creating a loop lateral to the internal carotid artery and then coursing posteriorly and medially to join the P1 segment of the posterior cerebral artery. The CP may also originate from the more medial undersurface of the internal carotid artery. The CP has a diameter that varies from 1 to 2.5 mm. Its complete absence is rare. The origins of the CP and the anterior choroidal artery are 3 to 4 mm apart. However, at the point where the CP joins the posterior cerebral artery, it is separated in a superior-inferior plane from the anterior choroidal artery by 1 cm or more. The CP can extend to 2 cm in length, and at times is tortuous before it joins the P1 segment of the posterior cerebral artery. There are from 3 to 12 perforators coursing superiorly and laterally from the CP. The first few millimeters of the CP from the internal carotid artery and the last few millimeters as it joins the P1 segment are the least likely areas to have perforators. The largest and most consistent perforator is the premammillary artery, which may be up to 1 mm in diameter. The premammillary artery usually originates from the middle third of the CP. It courses up in a superior and lateral direction, penetrating lateral to the mammillary body, in front of the peduncle and medial to the optic tract. It pierces this triangle to supply the lateral and medial anterior thalamic region. On rare occasions, perforators may originate from the junction of the posterior communicating artery and the P1 segment coursing into the interpeduncular fossa. Even if the CP is hypoplastic, it always has a distinct premammillary artery. Other smaller perforators from the PC go to the mammillary body, tuber cinereum, and peduncle

## 5.2 Anterior Choroidal Artery

The anterior choroidal artery (Ah) originates from the inferior lateral wall of the internal carotid artery, usually 3 to 4 mm distal to the origin of the posterior communicating artery. Absence of the Ah is rare. It may originate very close to the bifurcation of the internal carotid artery or at an almost common origin with the posterior communicating artery. However, the authors have found that a discrete origin of the Ah from the internal carotid artery is the rule rather than the exception. The artery itself can be as small as 0.5 mm and is rarely larger than 1.5 mm. At times, there are separate perforators originating simultaneously with the Ah or a separate branch of the Ah going to the medial temporal lobe and uncus. Careful dissection of the course of the Ah may yield up to 16 to 20 separate branches extending along its course. At its origin, the artery courses posteriorly 4 to 5 mm and then turns abruptly medial to the optic tract. It proceeds posteriorly and then laterally around the peduncle.

As the Ah courses posteriorly, it runs in the choroidal fissure. The choroidal fissure is a **C**-shaped structure that is ventrally concave from the point of the foramen of Monro; it extends posterior and inferior to end anteriorly in the temporal horn. The choroidal fissure is the site of the attachment of the choroid plexus in the lateral ventricles to the thalamus and fornix. The choroid plexus itself is attached to the fornix by the taenia fornicis and to the thalamus by the taenia choroidea (thalami). In the temporal horn, the taenia fornicis becomes the taenia fimbriae. The taeniae are small, membranous ridges in the choroidal fissure composed of one layer of pia mater and one layer of ependyma. A taenia has no neural tissue. The choroid plexus is surrounded by the ependymal layer as well.

The Ah terminates in the temporal horn of the lateral ventricle to supply the choroid plexus of the temporal horn and the atrium. Frequently, the Ah is proportionately larger if the posterior lateral choroidal blood supply is relatively small.

At the junction of the optic tract entering the lateral geniculate body, the Ah turns laterally and superiorly, giving branches to the lateral geniculate body. As the artery courses underneath and medial to the optic tract, it gives off branches both medially above the optic tract and laterally around it, penetrating the midbrain above. Some branches pierce the optic tract itself, supplying deeper structures, such as the globus pallidus and posterior limb of the internal capsule. The Ah also contributes to supplying the red nucleus and substantia nigra. The Ah and its branches and the posterior communicating artery with its perforators are draped in a common arachnoid veil.

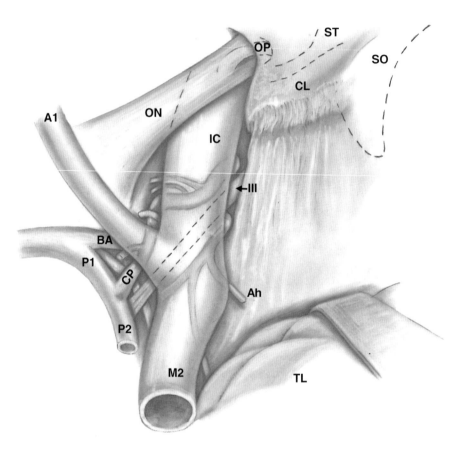

**Fig. 5.1** A view of the region of the supraclinoid internal carotid artery as seen through a right pterional craniotomy.

A1  anterior cerebral artery
Ah  anterior choroidal artery
BA  basilar artery
CL  anterior clinoid
CP  posterior communicating artery
IC  internal carotid artery
III  third nerve
M2  middle cerebral artery
ON  optic nerve
OP  ophthalmic artery
P1  posterior cerebral artery
P2  posterior cerebral artery
SO  superior orbital fissure
ST  optic strut
TL  temporal lobe

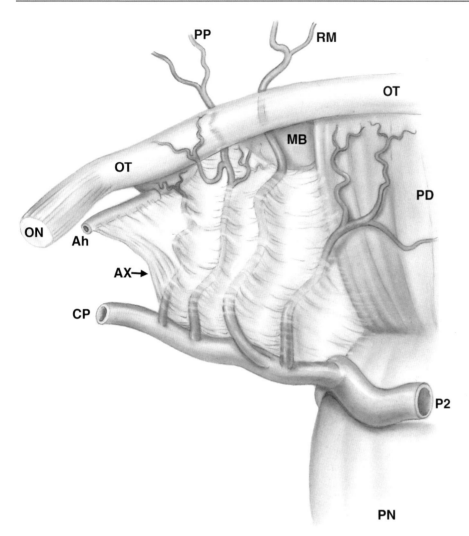

**Fig. 5.2** A left lateral view of the posterior communicating artery and its perforators. Note the common arachnoid veil (AX) between anterior choroidal artery (Ah) and posterior communicating artery (CP).

Ah   anterior choroidal artery
AX   arachnoid
CP   posterior communicating artery
MB   mammillary body
ON   optic nerve
OT   optic tract
PD   peduncle
PN   pons
PP   perforator to midbrain
P2   posterior cerebral artery
RM   premammillary artery

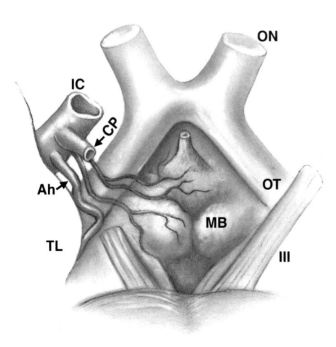

**Fig. 5.3** A ventral view of the brain illustrating the relationship between the posterior communicating artery and the anterior choroidal artery as they arise from the internal carotid artery.

Ah   anterior choroidal artery
CP   posterior communicating artery
IC   internal carotid artery
MB   mammillary body
ON   optic nerve
OT   optic tract
TL   temporal lobe
III   third nerve

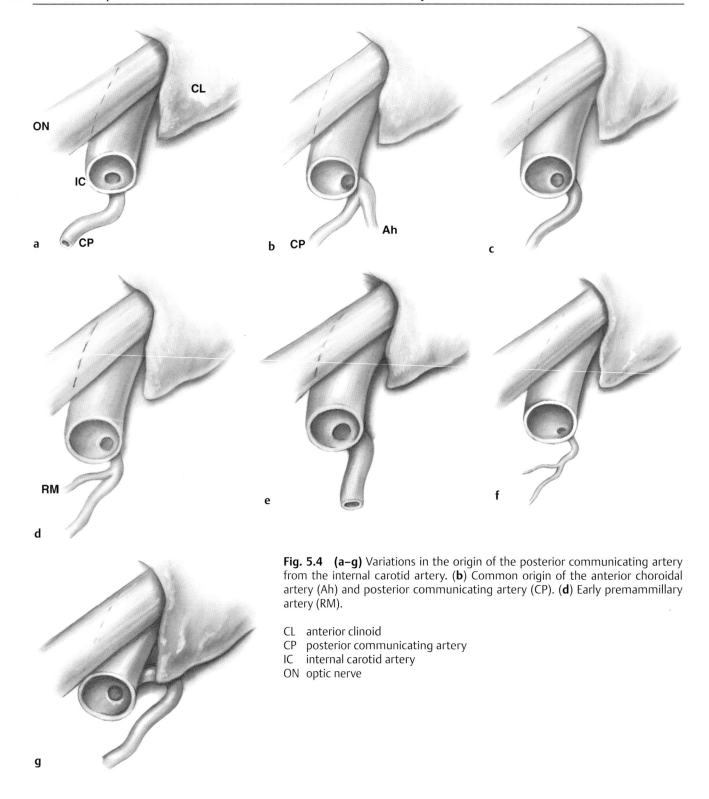

**Fig. 5.4 (a–g)** Variations in the origin of the posterior communicating artery from the internal carotid artery. (**b**) Common origin of the anterior choroidal artery (Ah) and posterior communicating artery (CP). (**d**) Early premammillary artery (RM).

CL anterior clinoid
CP posterior communicating artery
IC internal carotid artery
ON optic nerve

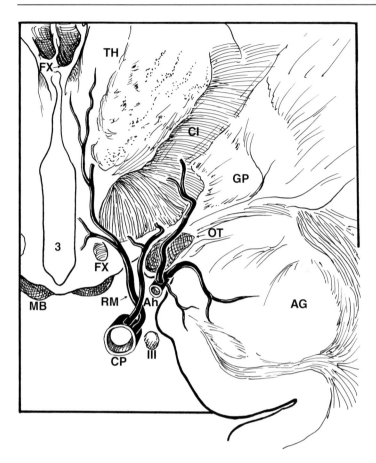

**Fig. 5.5**   A coronal view just in front of the mammillary bodies showing the relationship of the posterior communicating artery (CP) and the anterior choroidal artery (Ah) to structures in the region.

Ah   anterior choroidal artery
AG   amygdala
CI   internal capsule
CP   posterior communicating artery
FX   fornix
GP   globus pallidus
MB   mammillary body
OT   optic tract
RM   premammillary artery
TH   thalamus
III   third nerve
3   third ventricle

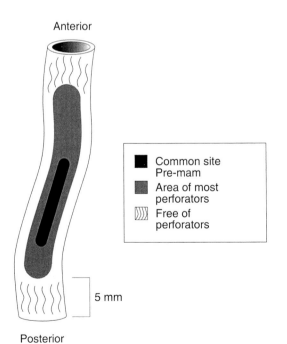

**Fig. 5.6**   Schematic of superior view of the posterior communicating artery. Although perforators can appear in the first 5 mm and last 5 mm of the posterior communicating artery, they are much less common. In addition, the premammillary artery can originate almost simultaneously with the posterior communicating artery on rare occasions.

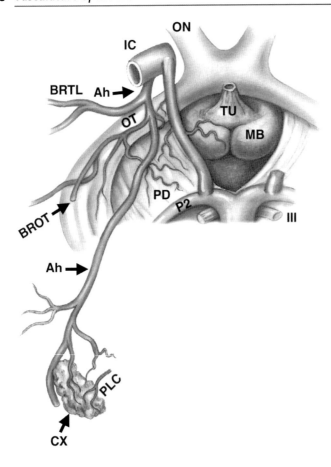

**Fig. 5.7** A ventral view of the brain showing the course of the anterior choroidal artery and its branches.

| | |
|---|---|
| Ah | anterior choroidal artery |
| BRTL | branch to temporal lobe |
| BROT | branch penetrating optic tract |
| CX | choroid plexus |
| IC | internal carotid artery |
| MB | mammillary body |
| ON | optic nerve |
| OT | optic tract |
| PD | peduncle |
| P2 | posterior cerebral artery |
| PLC | posterior lateral choroidal artery |
| TU | tuber cinereum |
| III | third nerve |

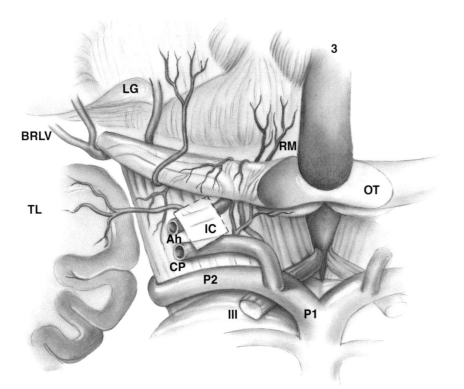

**Fig. 5.8** An anteroposterior (AP) view of the anterior choroidal artery and posterior communicating artery and the pattern of distribution of the perforators from these vessels. The cerebral hemisphere is shown in coronal section. This is similar to a view in an AP angiogram.

| | |
|---|---|
| Ah | anterior choroidal artery |
| BRLV | branch to lateral ventricle |
| IC | internal carotid artery |
| CP | posterior communicating artery |
| LG | lateral geniculate body |
| OT | optic tract |
| P1 | posterior cerebral artery |
| P2 | posterior cerebral artery |
| RM | premammillary artery |
| TL | temporal lobe |
| III | third nerve |
| 3 | third ventricle |

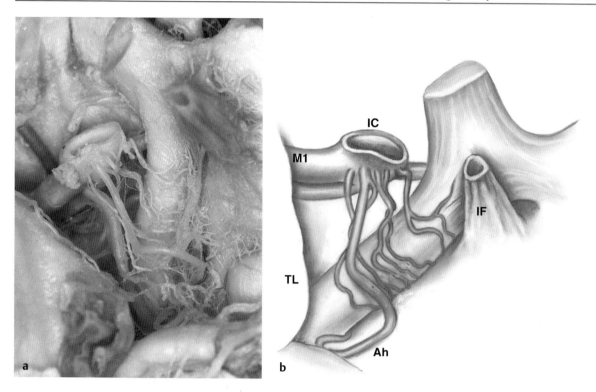

**Fig. 5.9   (a,b)** A ventral view of the region of the right optic tract. This shows the complex perforator pattern that may accompany the origin of the anterior choroidal artery. Note the anterior choroidal artery passing from lateral to medial inferior to the optic tract.

Ah   anterior choroidal artery
IC   internal carotid artery
IF   infundibulum
M1   middle cerebral artery
TL   temporal lobe

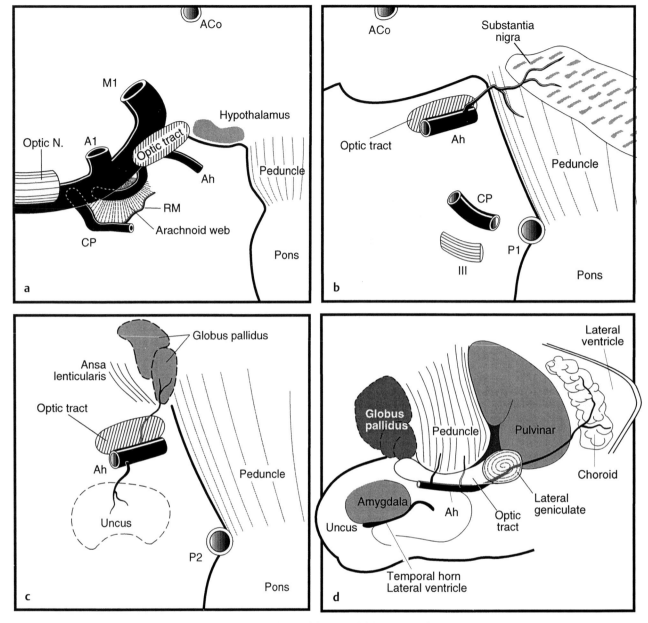

**Fig. 5.10 (a–d)** A medial view of the right anterior choroidal artery (Ah) in sagittal section proceeding laterally.

ACo  anterior commissure
Ah  anterior choroidal artery
A1  anterior cerebral artery
CP  posterior communicating artery
III  third nerve
M1  middle cerebral artery
P1  posterior cerebral artery
P2  posterior cerebral artery
RM  premammillary artery

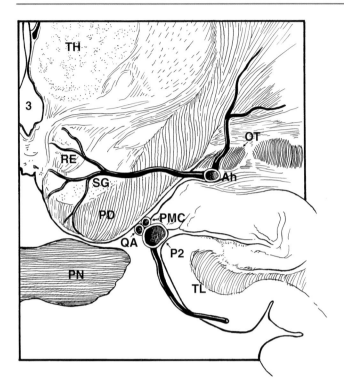

**Fig. 5.11**  A coronal section at the level of the red nucleus (RE). Note the perforator from the anterior choroidal artery piercing the peduncle and sending branches to the substantia nigra and red nucleus.

| | |
|---|---|
| Ah | anterior choroidal artery |
| OT | optic tract |
| P2 | posterior cerebral artery |
| PD | peduncle |
| PMC | posterior medial choroidal artery |
| PN | pons |
| QA | quadrigeminal artery |
| RE | red nucleus |
| SG | substantia nigra |
| TH | thalamus |
| TL | temporal lobe |
| 3 | third ventricle |

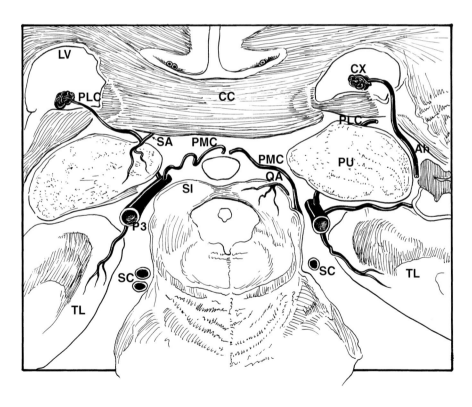

**Fig. 5.12**  A coronal section of the brain through the level of the pulvinar and the splenium of the corpus callosum. Note the common branch coming from the P3 segment of the posterior cerebral artery, which then divides into the splenial artery and the posterior lateral choroidal artery (left side of figure).

| | |
|---|---|
| Ah | anterior choroidal artery |
| CC | corpus callosum |
| CX | choroid plexus |
| LV | lateral ventricles |
| P3 | posterior cerebral artery |
| PLC | posterior lateral choroidal artery |
| PMC | posterior medial choroidal artery |
| PU | pulvinar |
| QA | quadrigeminal artery |
| SA | splenial artery |
| SC | superior cerebellar artery |
| TL | temporal lobe |
| SI | superior colliculus |

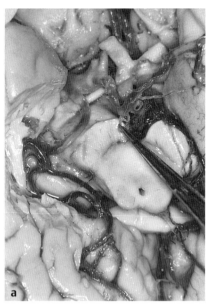

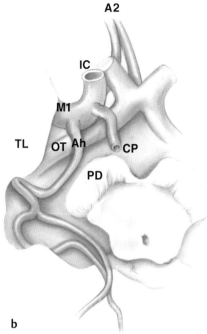

**Fig. 5.13** **(a,b)** A rare variant whereby the anterior choroidal artery becomes the main blood supply to the occipital lobe, including the calcarine cortex.

Ah  anterior choroidal artery
A2  anterior cerebral artery
CP  posterior communicating artery
IC  internal carotid artery
M1  middle cerebral artery
OT  optic tract
PD  peduncle
TL  temporal lobe

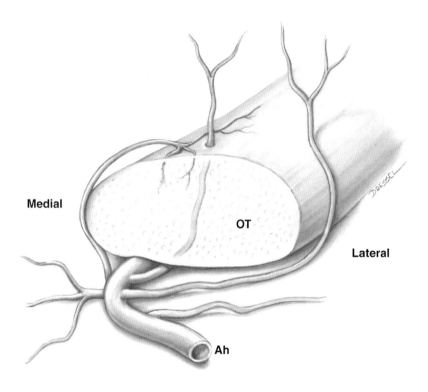

**Fig. 5.14** A composite illustration of the various relationships of the branches of the anterior choroidal artery to the optic tract. Note that perforators can pass directly through the optic tract and, in particular, supply the internal capsule and the globus pallidus. Also note that the direct blood supply to the optic tract from the anterior choroidal artery is usually a perforator that passes medially and then around the optic tract to penetrate superiorly.

Ah  anterior choroidal artery
OT  optic tract

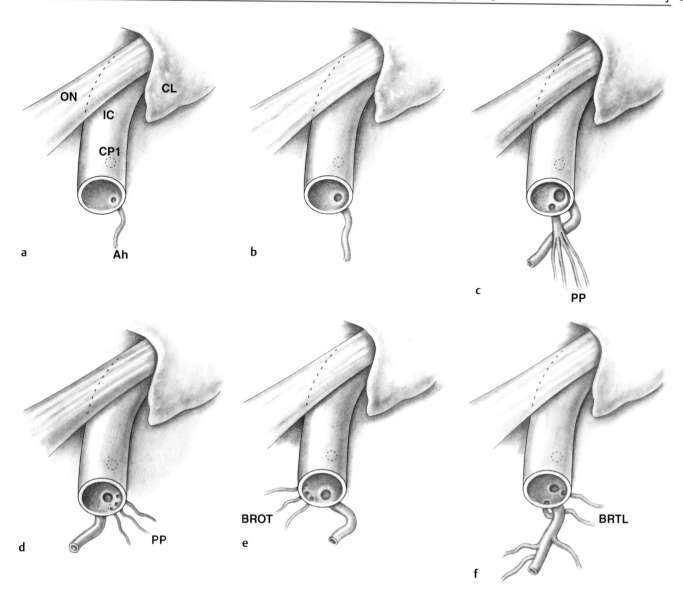

**Fig. 5.15 (a–f)** Variations of the anterior choroidal artery origin from the internal carotid artery. The origins of the anterior choroidal artery and posterior communicating artery are usually 4–5 mm apart, but can have a common origin.

Ah    anterior choroidal artery
CL    anterior clinoid
CP1   posterior communicating artery origin
IC    internal carotid artery
ON    optic nerve
PP    perforators
BRTL  branch to temporal lobe
BROT  branches to optic tract

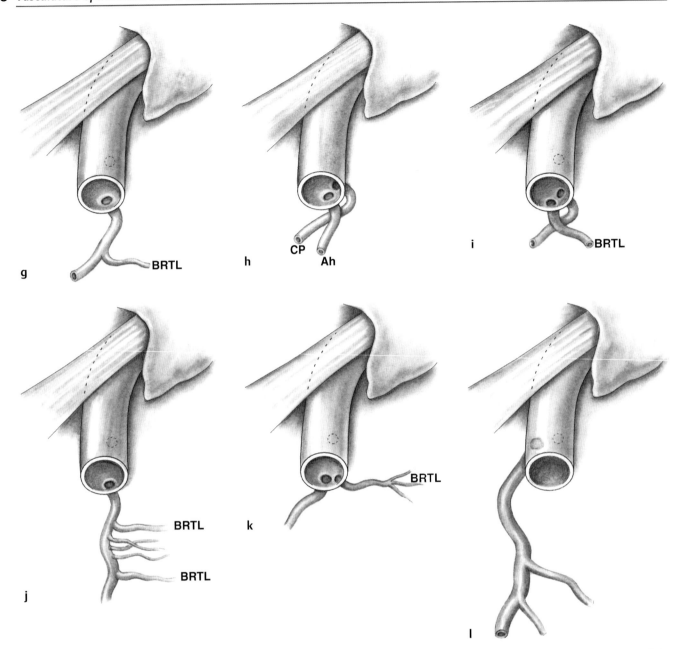

**Fig. 5.15** (*Continued*) **(g–l)** Variations of the anterior choroidal artery origin from the internal carotid artery. The origins of the anterior choroidal artery and posterior communicating artery are usually 4–5 mm apart, but can have a common origin.

Ah    anterior choroidal artery
BRTL  branch to temporal lobe
CP    posterior communicating artery

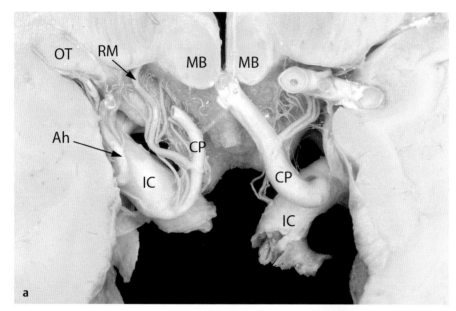

**Fig. 5.16** **(a)** Posterior-anterior view at the base of the brain showing each posterior communicating artery (CP) arising from the internal carotid arteries (IC).

MB mammillary body
RM premammillary artery
Ah anterior choroidal artery
OT optic tract

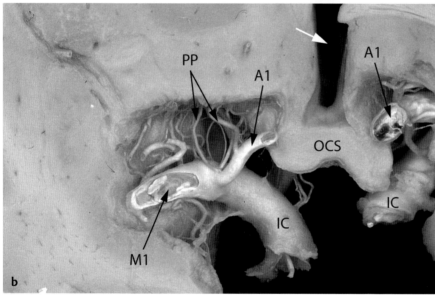

**Fig. 5.16** **(b)** Anterior-posterior view of **(a)**.

OCS optic chiasm
A1 anterior cerebral artery
IC internal carotid artery
M1 middle cerebral artery
PP perforators
White arrow third ventricle

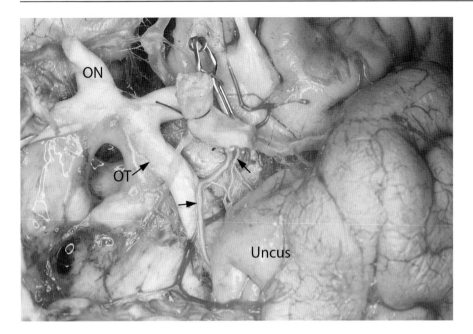

**Fig. 5.17** Ventral view of left hemisphere with selective injection of anterior choroidal artery (*left arrow*). Note separate branch (*right arrow*) from internal carotid artery to uncus.

OT  optic tract
ON  optic nerve

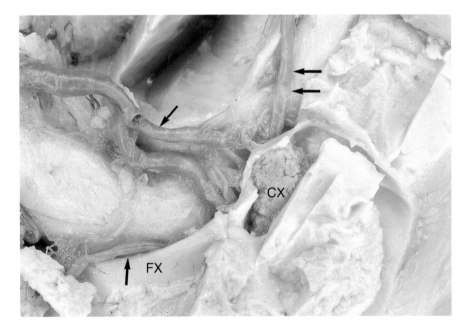

**5.18** Relationship of anterior choroidal artery, posterior lateral choroidal artery, and draining veins into basal vein of Rosenthal.

⇐  anterior choroidal artery
↑  posterior lateral choroidal artery (PLC)
↓  basal vein of Rosenthal
CX  choroid plexus
FX  fornix

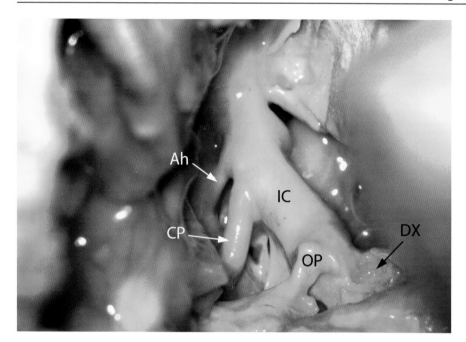

**Fig. 5.19** View of the right intradural internal carotid artery (IC).

DX distal ring
OP ophthalmic artery
CP posterior communicating artery
Ah anterior choroidal artery

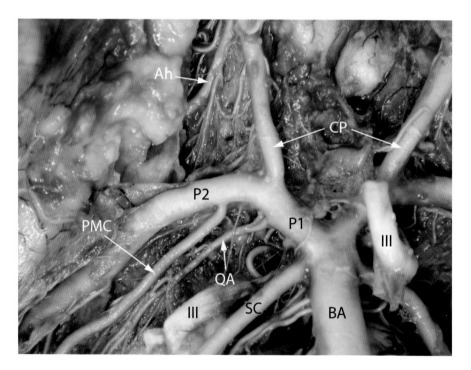

**Fig. 5.20** Ventral view of basilar bifurcation.

Ah anterior choroidal artery
BA basilar artery
SC superior cerebellar artery
CP posterior communicating artery
QA quadrigeminal artery
PMC posterior medial choroidal artery
P1, P2 posterior cerebral artery
III third nerve

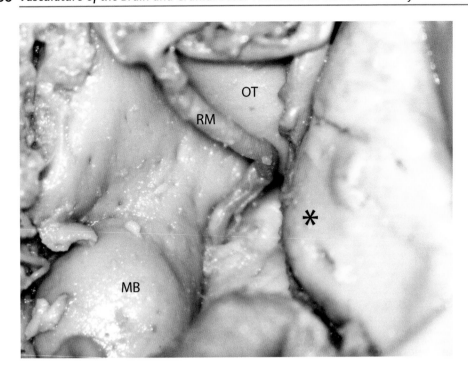

**Fig. 5.21** Close-up ventral view of the premammillary artery (RM).

MB  mammillary body
OT  optic tract
*   uncus

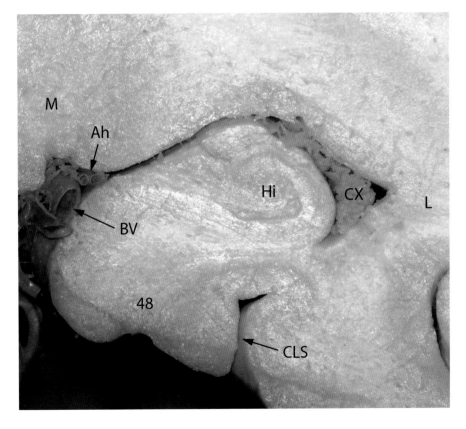

**Fig. 5.22** Cross section through the midtemporal lobe.

M    medial
L    lateral
BV   basal vein of Rosenthal
Hi   hippocampus
48   parahippocampal gyrus
Ah   anterior choroidal artery
CX   choroid plexus
CLS  collateral sulcus

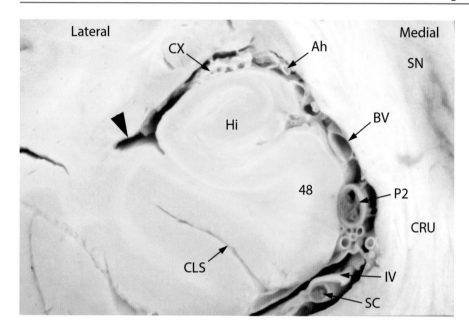

**Fig. 5.23**   Cross section through mid-temporal lobe.

Arrowhead   ventricle (temporal horn)
Ah   anterior choroidal artery
P2   posterior cerebral artery
SC   superior cerebellar artery
IV   fourth nerve
BV   basal vein of Rosenthal
Hi   hippocampus
48   parahippocampus
CLS   collateral fissure
CRU   crus cerebri
SN   substancia nigra
CX   choroid plexus

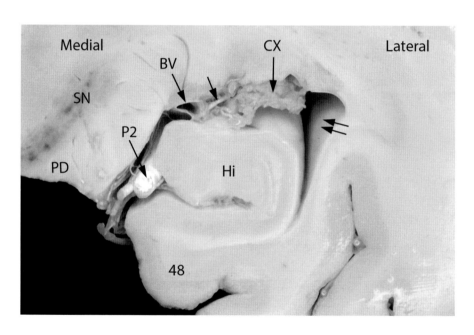

**Fig. 5.24**   Cross section through temporal lobe.

Arrow   choroidal fissure (membrane)
Double arrow   temporal horn
CX   choroid plexus
Hi   hippocampus
P2   posterior cerebral artery
48   parahippocampal gyrus
BV   basal vein of Rosenthal
PD   peduncle
SN   substancia nigra

## 5.3 Clinical Cases

### 5.3.1 Case 1

A middle-aged woman presented with a transient ischemic attack causing transient left hemiparesis. Computed tomographic angiography suggested a distal posterior communicating (PCom) aneurysm, which was noted on angiography to be a distal anterior choroidal artery (Ah) aneurysm. Given the small caliber of the Ah and the wide neck of the aneurysm, the patient was taken for a right orbitozygomatic craniotomy. After a wide Sylvian exposure and identification of the Ah, the medical uncus was subpially resected and the aneurysm found immediately posterior to the uncus. Clip reconstruction allowed preservation of the large Ah trunk. The patient tolerated the procedure without any neurological deficits.

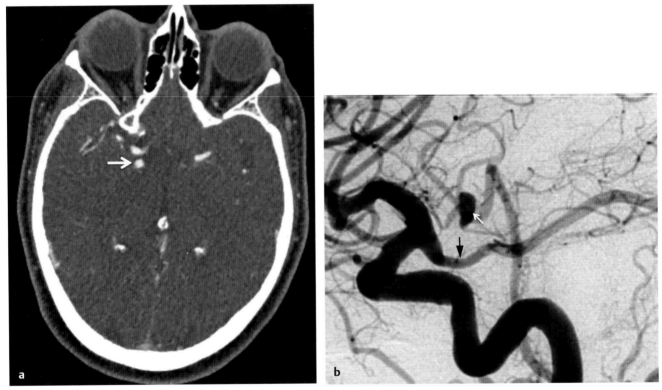

**Fig. 5.25** **(a)** A computed tomographic angiogram of the head. A right distal anterior choroidal artery aneurysm (*arrow*). **(b)** Right internal carotid artery angiogram. The aneurysm (*white arrow*) arises from the trunk of the anterior choroidal artery. Posterior communicating artery (*black arrow*).

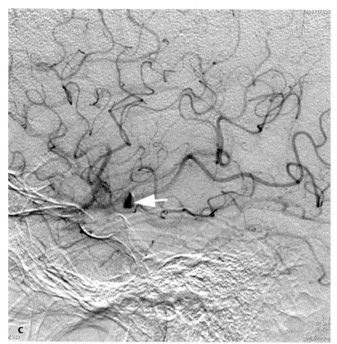

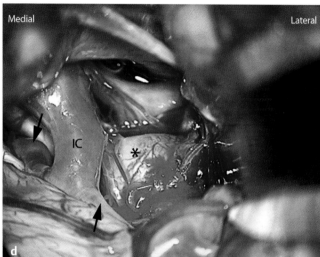

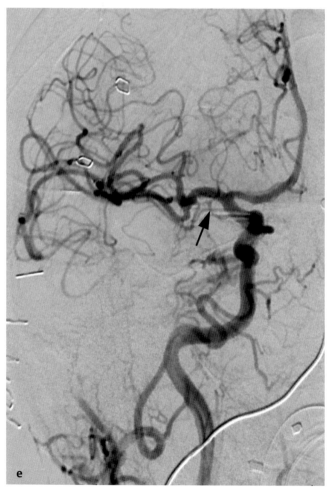

**Fig. 5.25** (*Continued*)  **(c)** Delayed phase from **(b)**. Stasis in the aneurysm (*arrow*). **(d)** Intraoperative photo at the right orbitozygomatic craniotomy shows the anterior choridal artery aneurysm (*asterisk*), right internal carotid artery (IC), M1 of the right middle cerebral artery (*right arrow*), and A1 of the right anterior cerebral artery (*left arrow*). **(e)** Intraoperative right internal carotid artery angiogram. The aneurysm has been clipped and obliterated with preservation of the anterior choroidal artery (*arrow*).

## 5.3.2 Case 2

A middle-aged man presented with pulsatile tinnitis, and magnetic resonance angiography was concerning for an intracranial aneurysm. The angiogram revealed the posterior communicating artery arising distal to the anterior choroidal artery. No aneurysm was found.

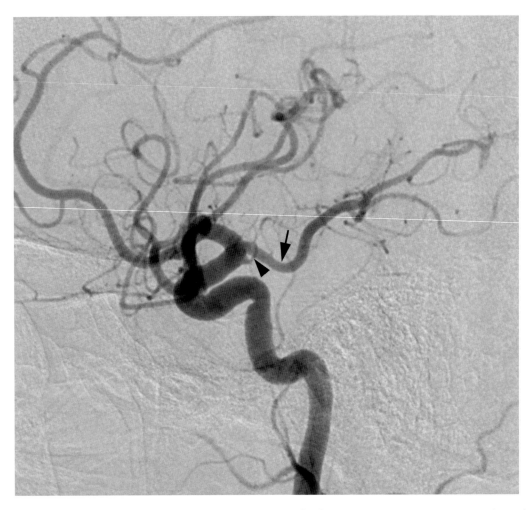

**Fig. 5.26** Lateral internal carotid angiogram. There is a fetal posterior communicating artery (*arrow*). As an incidental anomaly, the anterior choroidal artery (*arrowhead*) arises proximal to the posterior communicating artery, rather than the usual distal origin.

### 5.3.3 Case 3

A middle-aged woman presented with headaches and intermittent double vision. Workup, including magnetic resonance imaging and magnetic resonance angiography, resulted in discovery of a giant left cavernous aneurysm. The angiogram confirmed the presence of a giant cavernous segment aneurysm. After consideration of all options, a flow diverter device was placed from the proximal supraclinoidal segment across the neck of the aneursym; however, after deployment and during retrieval of the stent delivery system, the flow diverter foreshortened and was displaced into the aneurysm. Multiple attempts at anterograde reaccess through the stent were futile. To attempt a retrograde reaccess, because the distal flow diverter was still secure in the supraclinoidal

artery, we established a second groin vascular access and catheterized the left vertebral artery. Using a microcatheter and microwire, we selectively catheterized the left PCom and through it gained access into the left supraclinoidal ICA, subsequently the stent until the microwire exited the proximal flow diverter. We then used a snare through yet another microcatheter to ensnare the trans-PCom microwire and pull the microcatheter anterogradely through the flow diverter until it was in the supraclinoidal ICA (dental floss technique). At this point, we loosened the microwire, removed the snare, and placed additional flow diverters to reconstruct the cavernous ICA. The patient made an excellent recovery, and diplopia and mass effect completely resolved.

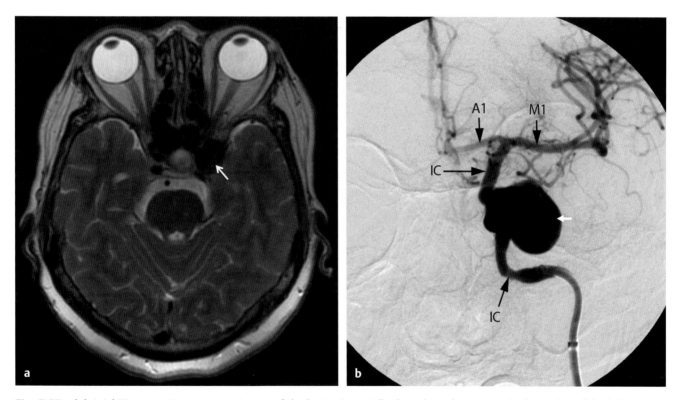

**Fig. 5.27   (a)** Axial T2 magnetic resonance image of the brain. A partially thrombosed aneurysm in the region of the left cavernous sinus (*arrow*). **(b)** Left internal carotid artery angiogram. Left internal carotid artery aneurysm (*arrow*) in the cavernous sinus.

IC   internal carotid artery
A1   anterior cerebral artery
M1   middle cerebral artery

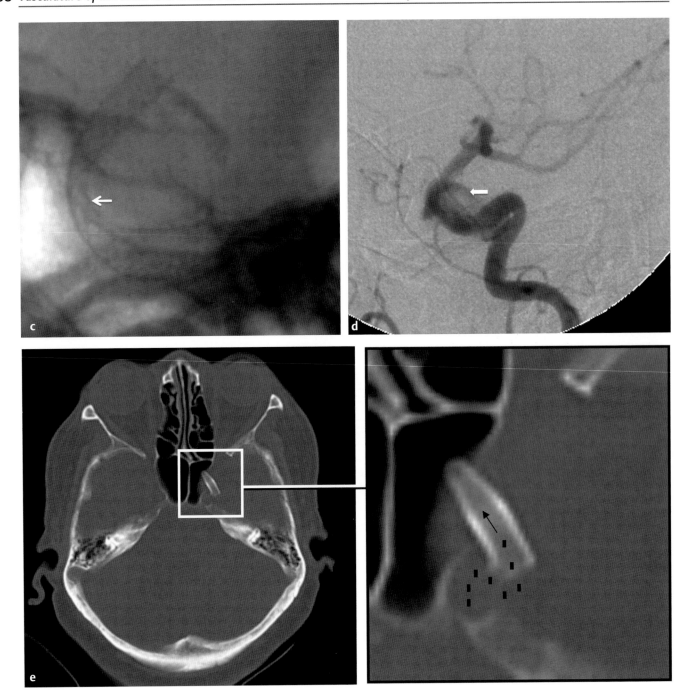

**Fig. 5.27** (*Continued*) **(c)** Intraprocedure endovascular fluoroscopic image of the head. An intravascular flow diverter has been deployed in the right internal carotid artery (*arrow*). **(d)** Right lateral internal carotid angiogram after deployment of the flow diverter stent. Stasis of contrast in the aneurysm (*arrow*). **(e)** Postendovascular intervention noncontrasted computed tomographic image of the head. There is foreshortening of the flow diverter (*box*) into the aneurysm. The arrow (enlargement of box) indicates flow into the diverter lumen from the aneurysm.

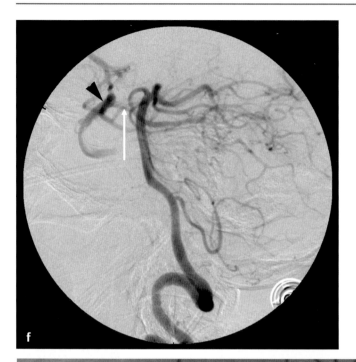

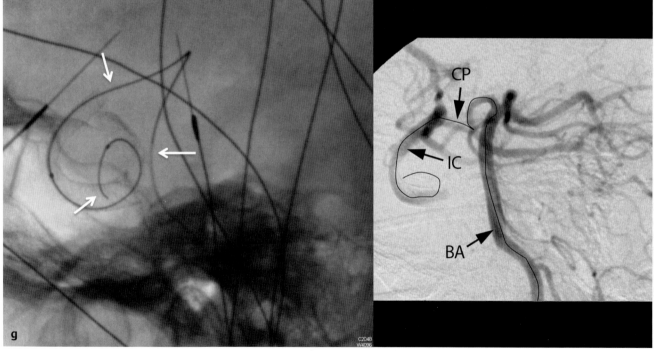

**Fig. 5.27** (*Continued*)   **(f)** Left vertebral angiogram. A large left posterior communicating artery is evident (*arrow*) communicating with the left internal carotid artery (*arrowhead*). **(g)** A microguidewire (*arrows on left*) is inserted inside the aneurysm. On the right it traverses the left vertebral (*not shown*) and basilar artery (BA) through the left posterior communicating artery (CP) into the left internal carotid artery (IC).

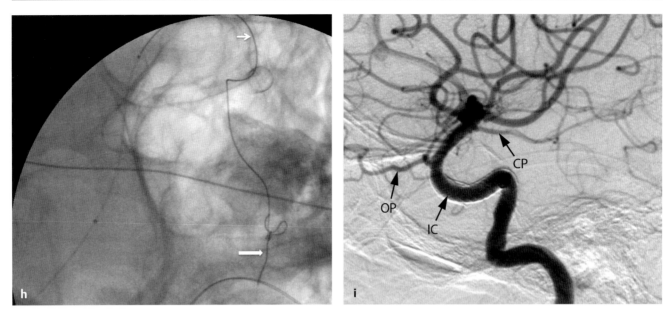

**Fig. 5.27** (*Continued*)   **(h)** Simultaneous with **(g)**, left transcarotid catheterization (*lower arrow*) of the aneurysm. A snare has grabbed the microwire (*upper arrow*) that was passed through the posterior communicating artery (CP) via the left vertebral artery. Additional flow diverters were then placed. **(i)** A postendovascular intervention left internal carotid angiogram at 6 months. The left internal carotid (IC) artery is completely reconstructed. The aneurysm does not fill.

OP   ophthalmic artery

## Clinical Pearls

- Prior to clipping a posterior communicating aneurysm, it is important to establish the relationship between the anterior clinoid process and the posterior communicating artery. If the posterior communicating artery arises more proximal than usual and underneath the anterior clinoid process, proximal vascular control may require cervical internal carotid artery exposure. In addition, it is also important when exposing a posterior communicating aneurysm not to retract the temporal lobe until the aneurysm has been completely exposed because the aneurysm may be tethered to the medial temporal lobe and tentorial dura, and rupture may occur during retraction before the arachnoid has been completely dissected.

- When one is clipping basilar terminus aneurysms, the posterior communicating artery (CP) may obstruct the needed view of the aneurysm neck and associated perforators. In cases where the CP is not fetal or large with a hypoplastic P1 segment, it can be sharply divided between two mini/arteriovenous malformation clips at its junction with the PCA. This is preferable to bipolar cautery, which invariably compromises the distal CP anterior thalamoperforators.

- When clipping posterior communicating artery aneurysms, it is critical to clearly identify the proximal anterior choroidal artery (Ah) because failure to do so may result in the posterior communicating clip compromising or occluding the main Ah, resulting in long-term hemiplegia.

- Endovascular catherization of the anterior choroidal artery, as may be considerd during embolization of pial arteriovenous malformations, is a much higher risk than other major named branches in the intracranial circulation. It should be treated essentially the same as lenticulostriate, thalamoperforators, or basilar trunk perforators. It is an end vessel, and either direct vascular injury or embolic material reflux in the parent vessel, as is frequently encountered, may pose the risk of major neurological deficits.

# 6 Middle Cerebral Artery

The middle cerebral artery originates at the terminal division of the internal carotid artery just at the level of the olfactory trigone and lateral to the optic chiasm. The artery then courses forward and laterally after passing over the limen insulae to enter the insula. The main bifurcation of the middle cerebral artery is variable. At times, the bifurcation will appear right at the limen insulae. However, if the M1 segment (the segment from the origin to the division of the artery) is quite elongated, the definitive bifurcation may not appear until the artery is actually within the insular region. After dividing, the main divisions and cortical branches of the middle cerebral artery course over the surface of the insula and then loop over the frontal, parietal, and temporal lobes to extend into the sulci of the surface of the brain. Branches may have to course up to 5 cm before emerging from the Sylvian fissure over the surface of the brain. The middle cerebral artery can have a defined bifurcation or trifurcation or variations in between. Given the variability of the distal branches of the middle cerebral artery, precise nomenclature of these vessels is problematic. However, one can divide the areas of distal branching into temporal (anterior temporal, midtemporal, posterior temporal), frontal (inferior, middle, posterior), central, parietal (supramarginal, angular), and temporo-occipital.

## 6.1 Anterior/Temporal

Frequently, the M1 segment will provide a separate anterior temporal branch prior to the M1 bifurcation or trifurcation. At times, an anterior temporal artery may originate from the internal carotid artery just prior to its bifurcation. Rather than a true "accessory middle cerebral artery," this is merely an early branch of the middle cerebral artery and supplies only the anterior temporal region. However, large perforators may arise from this relatively small branch. A true accessory middle cerebral artery originates from the A2 segment of the anterior cerebral artery and courses laterally, entering the Sylvian fissure parallel to the middle cerebral artery and supplying the frontal cortex.

## 6.2 Frontal

The frontal branches of the middle cerebral artery consist of the orbital frontal, the ascending frontal or middle frontal branch, and the precentral or posterior frontal branch. At times, the central and precentral arteries have a common origin. The configuration of the frontal branches is somewhat dependent on whether the central artery originates frontally or more distally.

The central sulcus artery may originate in conjunction with the frontal branches or in common with the supramarginal–angular complex. At times, this artery is double or bifurcates and may overlap with the blood supply of the postcentral artery and precentral artery. The central artery courses in the rolandic fissure.

## 6.3 Parietal

The parietal distribution of the middle cerebral artery consists of blood supply to the postcentral gyrus and the supramarginal and angular gyri. The configuration is dependent on how the middle cerebral artery bifurcates or trifurcates. In general, the artery that ultimately supplies the angular gyrus courses over Heschl's gyrus. At times, a small supplementary artery from the temporo-occipital branch contributes to the angular supply. The central artery may originate from the supramarginal branch itself.

## 6.4 Temporo-occipital

The temporo-occipital division of the middle cerebral artery may supply the entire temporal lobe, as well as extend quite posteriorly into the lateral occipital lobe, contributing to its blood supply. The temporo-occipital branch may be an early, very distinct, large-caliber branch originating deep in the Sylvian fissure and extending quite a distance posteriorly. As it courses posteriorly, it gives branches to the anterior, midtemporal, and posterior temporal regions. It may also contribute a separate branch posteriorly to the angular gyrus. At times, the temporo-occipital branch is attenuated and originates in common with the other parietal branches. In this case, the anterior temporal region and midtemporal region may be supplied by separate branches from the M1 segment.

## 6.5 Perforator Patterns of the Middle Cerebral Artery

The lenticulostriate perforating arteries arise from the superior portion of the middle cerebral artery (M1) and supply the substantia innominata, the lateral portion of the anterior commissure, the putamen, the lateral segment of the globus pallidus, the superior half of the internal capsule and the adjacent corona radiata, and the body and head of the caudate nucleus. There are medial and lateral striate arteries. The patterns of the perforators arising from the middle cerebral artery vary. They can be divided into three patterns: (1) large perforators predominate in the most proximal half of the middle cerebral artery (M1) before its major division, (2) large perforators predominate in the most distal half of the M1 before its major division, and (3) large perforators are seen in the M2 branches of the middle cerebral artery after its major division.

Typically, the perforators very close to the bifurcation of the internal carotid artery are of smaller caliber. The length of the M1 segment of the middle cerebral artery does not necessarily coincide with any pattern of perforators.

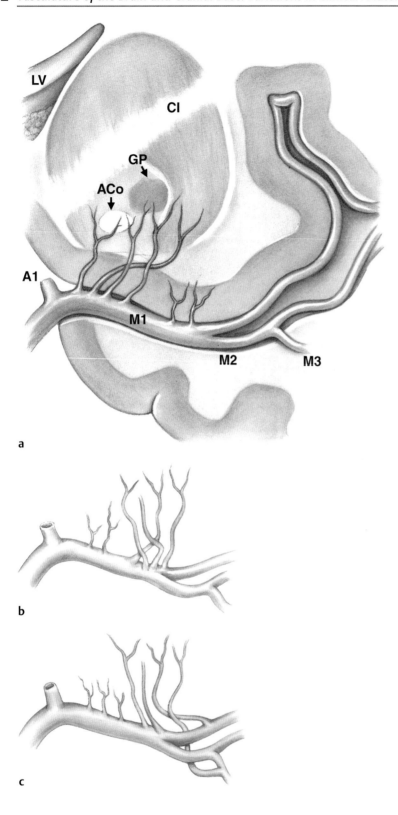

a

b

c

**Fig. 6.1** **(a–c)** Coronal section through the left hemisphere at the level of the anterior commissure showing the three basic configurations of the perforator patterns from the proximal middle cerebral artery. Note **(c)** where perforators arise from the M2 and M3 segments.

A1   anterior cerebral artery
ACo anterior commissure
CI    internal capsule
GP   globus pallidus
LV    lateral ventricle
M1   middle cerebral artery
M2   middle cerebral artery
M3   middle cerebral artery

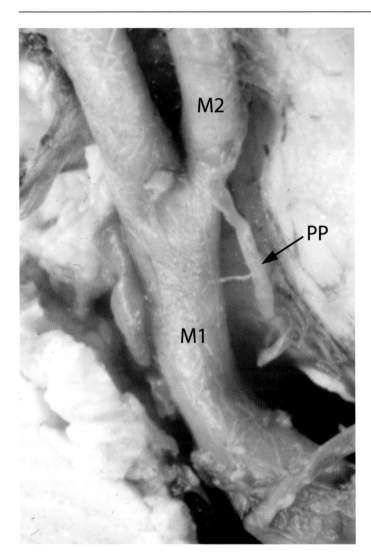

**Fig. 6.2** A large perforator (PP) of the middle cerebral artery (M2 segment) passing retrograde.

M1 proximal middle cerebral artery

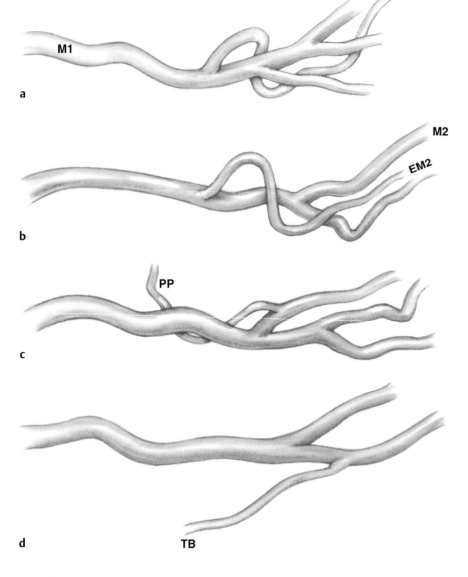

**Fig. 6.3 (a–d)** Variations of the branching of the M1 segment of the middle cerebral artery.

M1   middle cerebral artery
M2   middle cerebral artery
EM2  early M2 branch to parietal region
PP   perforator
TB   temporal artery branch (anterior)

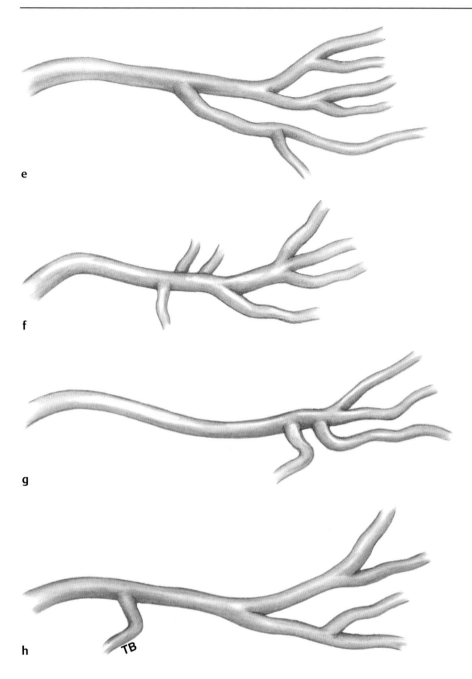

**Fig. 6.3 (e–h)** Variations of the branching of the M1 segment of the middle cerebral artery.

TB   temporal artery branch (anterior)

e

f

g

h   TB

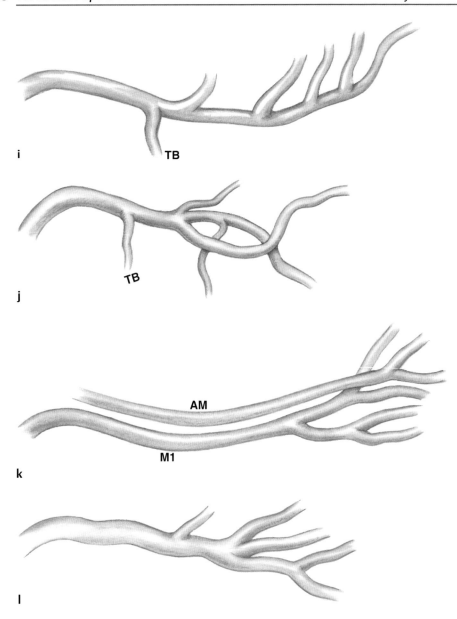

**Fig. 6.3 (i–l)** Variations of the branching of the M1 segment of the middle cerebral artery.

AM  accessory middle cerebral artery from A2
M1  middle cerebral artery
TB  temporal artery branch (anterior)

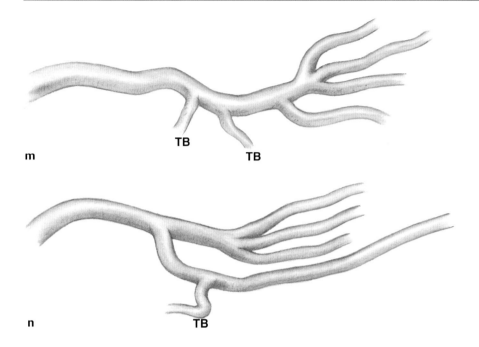

**Fig. 6.3 (m,n)** Variations of the branching of the M1 segment of the middle cerebral artery.

TB temporal artery branch (anterior)

m

n

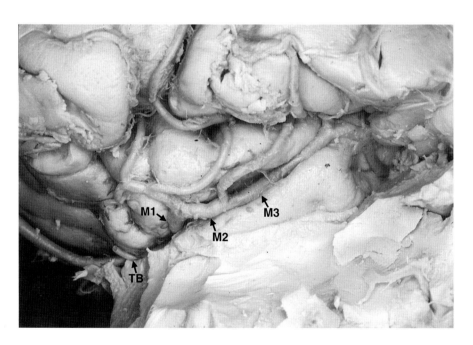

**Fig. 6.4** M1 bifurcation pattern similar to that in **Figs. 6.3h** and **6.3l**.

M1 middle cerebral artery
M2 middle cerebral artery
M3 middle cerebral artery
TB temporal artery branch (anterior)

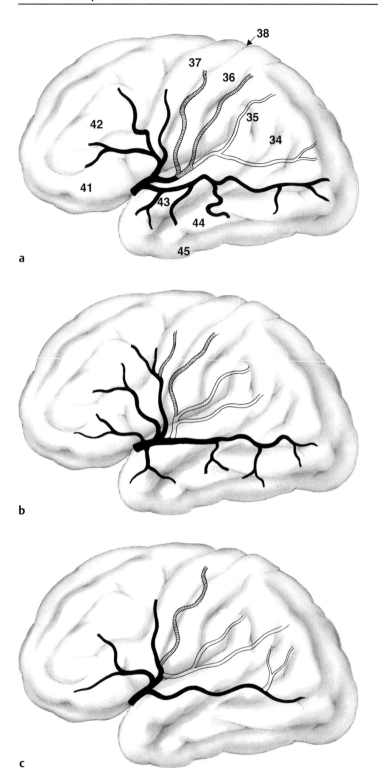

a

b

c

**Fig. 6.5** Patterns of distribution of the distal branch of the middle cerebral artery. **(a–g)** The central, supramarginal, and angular originate from a common stem. There is a large separate temporal branch. **(h–l)** The central artery has a frontal origin. **(m–r)** A mixed variation, but more typical is a separate vessel to angular gyrus from a large temporal artery. **(s,t)** The central, supramarginal, angular, and temporal originate as a "three-way split." **(u)** Accessory middle cerebral artery (AM) originates from A2, supplies the frontal region, and gives off the central artery. (See **Figs. 6.3k** and **7.3i**.)

☐ supramarginal and angular branches
▨ central artery(ies)
■ frontal and/or temporo-occipital branches
34 angular gyrus
35 supramarginal gyrus
36 postcentral gyrus
37 precentral gyrus
38 central sulcus (fissure)
41 inferior frontal gyrus
42 middle frontal gyrus
43 superior temporal gyrus
44 middle temporal gyrus
45 inferior temporal gyrus

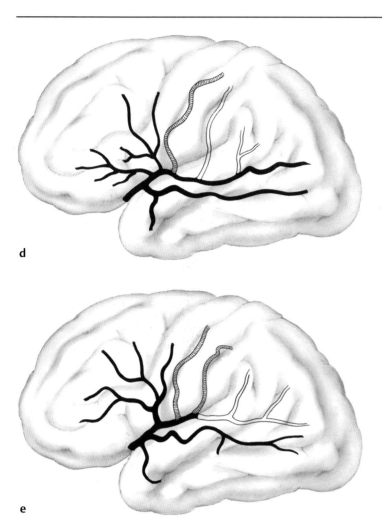

d

e

**Fig. 6.5**   Patterns of distribution of the distal branch of the middle cerebral artery. **(d,e)** The central, supramarginal, and angular originate from common stem.

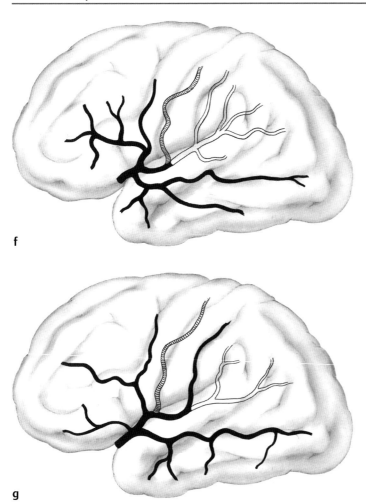

f

g

**Fig. 6.5** Patterns of distribution of the distal branch of the middle cerebral artery. **(f,g)** Similar to **(a–e)**.

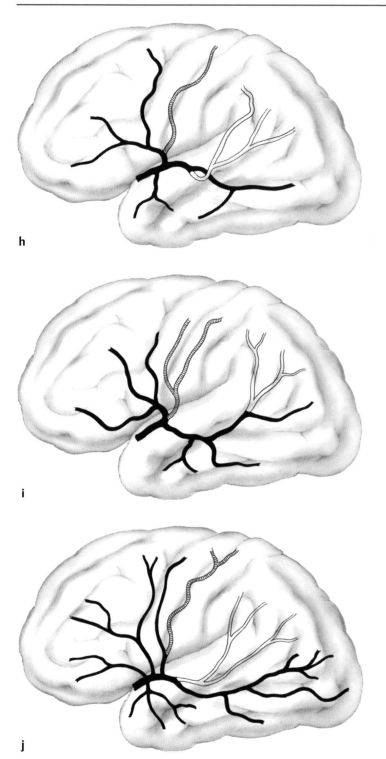

h

i

j

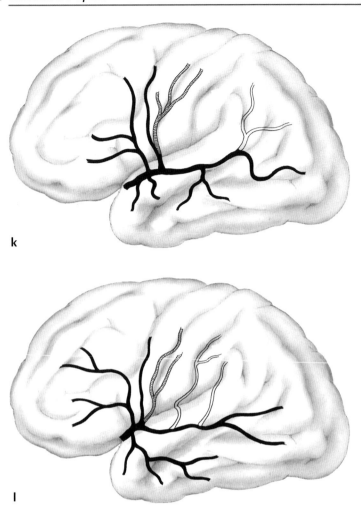

k

l

**Fig. 6.5** Patterns of distribution of the distal branch of the middle cerebral artery. **(k,l)** The central artery has a frontal origin.

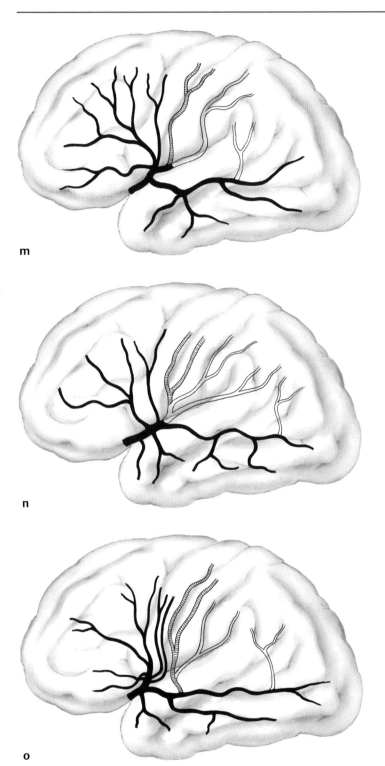

m

n

o

**Fig. 6.5** Patterns of distribution of the distal branch of the middle cerebral artery. **(m–o)** Separate angular artery from large temporal vessel.

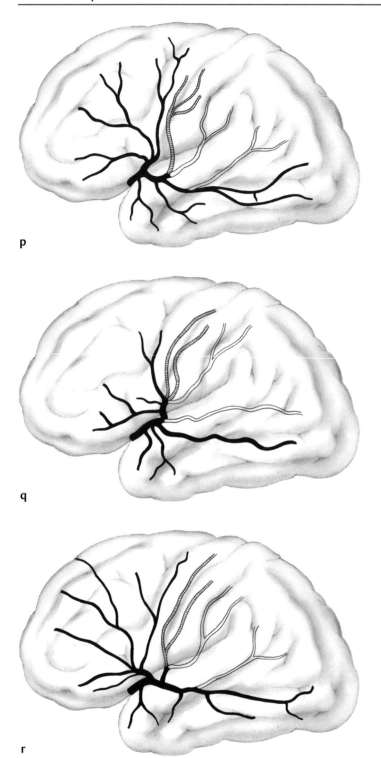

**Fig. 6.5** Patterns of distribution of the distal branch of the middle cerebral artery. **(p–r)** Similar to **(m–o)**.

p

q

r

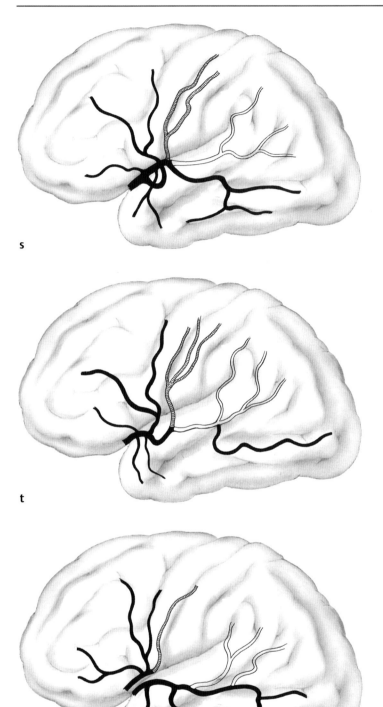

s

t

u

**Fig. 6.5** Patterns of distribution of the distal branch of the middle cerebral artery. **(s,t)** "Three-way split" of central, supramarginal, and angular.

**Fig. 6.5** Patterns of distribution of the distal branch of the middle cerebral artery. **(u)** True accessory middle cerebral artery.

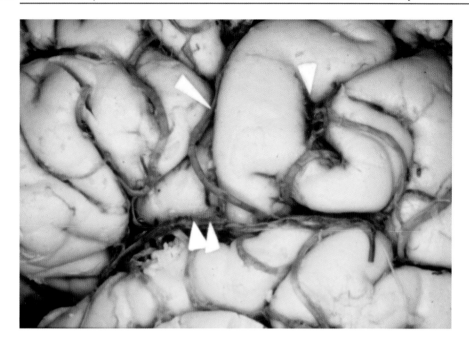

**Fig. 6.6** Precentral artery (*upper left arrowhead*). Central sulcus with two arteries entering (*upper right arrowhead*). Superficial middle cerebral vein (*double arrowheads*).

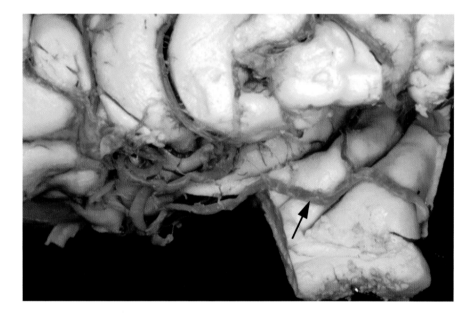

**Fig. 6.7** Branch of the middle cerebral artery (*arrow*) coursing over Heschl's gyrus. This branch frequently gives rise to the angular artery.

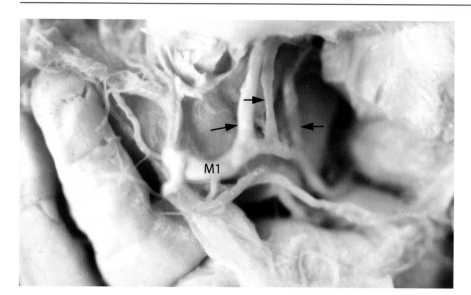

**Fig. 6.8** Trifurcation (*three arrows*) of M1.

M1 proximal middle cerebral artery

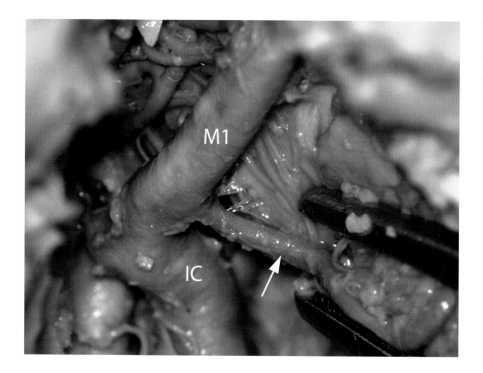

**Fig. 6.9** Early temporal branch (*arrow*) from the middle cerebral artery (M1).

IC internal carotid artery

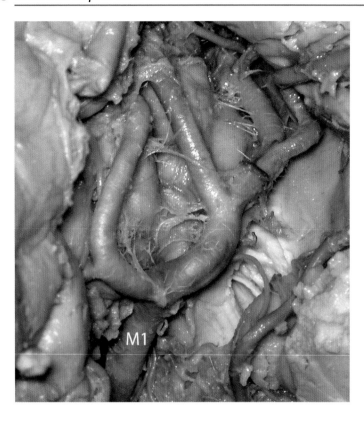

**Fig. 6.10** The middle cerebral artery (M1) with sequential large caliber bifurcations.

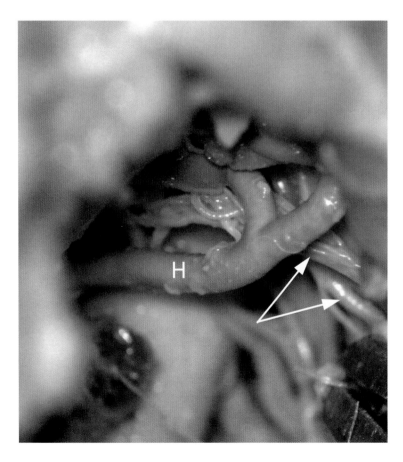

**Fig. 6.11** Heubner's artery (H) bifurcates as it terminates just medial to the lateral striate branches (*two arrows*) of the middle cerebral artery.

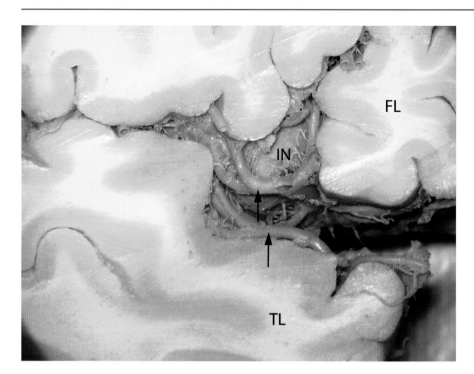

**Fig. 6.12** Sagittal section of right hemisphere, exposing Sylvian fissure and middle cerebral artery complex (*arrows*).

IN  insula
TL  temporal lobe
FL  frontal lobe

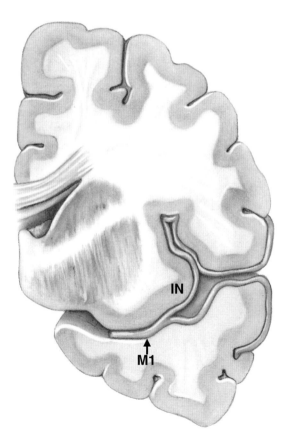

**Fig. 6.13** Coronal section through left hemisphere showing the contour of the middle cerebral artery in the insula and emergence over the surface of convexity of hemisphere.

IN  insula
M1  middle cerebral artery

## 6.6 Clinical Cases

### 6.6.1 Case 1

A middle-aged man presented with right hemiparesis and severe headaches. Computed tomographic scan demonstrated a giant, partially thrombosed M1 segment aneurysm. The angiogram revealed a small component that was filling along a large lateral lenticulostriate vessel. The saccular component was coiled, leaving enough of a proximal pouch to continue supply to the lateral lenticulostriate, and a single flow diverter was placed across the M1 segment. Delayed angiography revealed complete obliteration of the aneurysm with a significant reduction in mass effect, resorption of the thrombosed aneurysm, and complete recovery of hemiparesis.

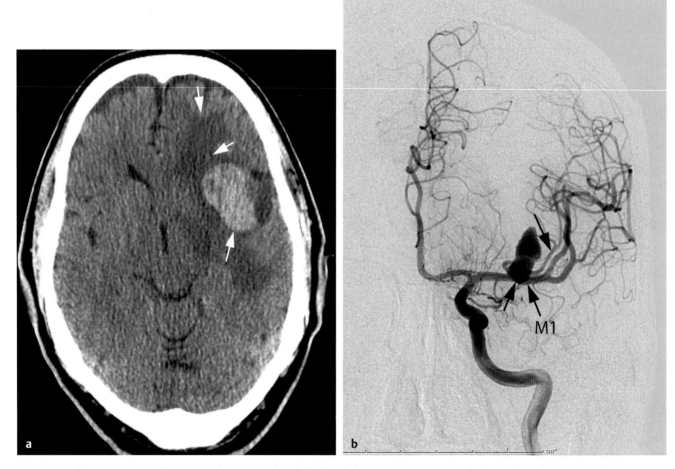

**Fig. 6.14** **(a)** Noncontrasted computed tomography of the head showing a giant, partially thrombosed aneurysm (*lower arrow*) with surrounding edema in the left frontal lobe (*upper arrows*). **(b)** Left internal carotid artery angiogram. There is a dilated pouch at the base of the aneurysm (*left arrow*) with an associated large, lateral lenticulostriate artery (*right upper arrow*). M1, middle cerebral artery.

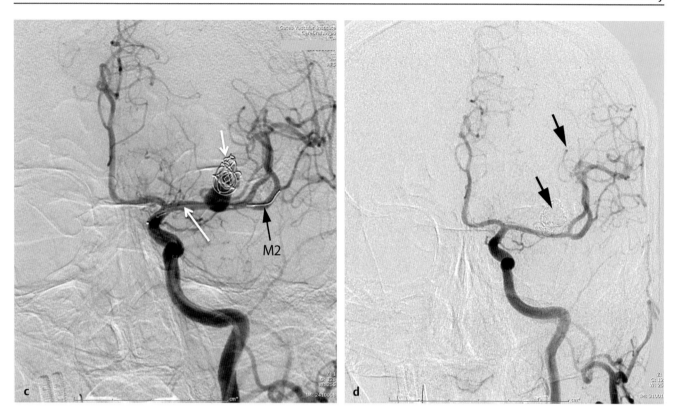

**Fig. 6.14** (*Continued*)   **(c)** A microcatheter (*left lower arrow*) was "jailed" inside the aneurysm sac, and a flow diverter was placed across the neck, ensuring no jailing of the M2 middle cerebral artery segment. Coils (*upper arrow*) were placed inside the aneurysm, leaving flow at the base of the aneurysm and allowing filling of the large lenticulostriate artery. **(d)** Delayed left internal carotid angiogram. Complete obliteration of the aneurysm (*lower arrow*) with coiling and diminished flow in the large lenticulostriate artery (*upper arrow*).

## 6.6.2 Case 2

An elderly man presented after being found upon wakening to have dense right hemiplegia and aphasia with a National Institutes of Health (NIH) stroke score of 20. His delay in presentation contraindicated intravenous thrombolytics. Computed tomographic (CT) angiography revealed a distal left M1 occlusion, and a CT perfusion scan suggested a large penumbra with a relatively small core. He was taken emergently for endovascular intervention. An angiogram confirmed a distal left M1 occlusion. A large-bore aspiration catheter was brought proximal to the clot into the M1 and then, through a microcatheter over a microwire, was used to cross the clot into the distal M2/3 segment.

After confirmation of the clot length, using a simultaneous angiogram from a microcatheter and proximal guide catheters, a stent retriever was delivered across the clot. The stent retriever was left open for about 5 minutes, allowing flow to the distal ischemic territory. Thereafter, aspiration was begun through the large-bore aspiration catheter, and the stent retriever was withdrawn entirely into the aspiration catheter. Repeat angiography revealed complete (TICI-3) revascularization. On the subsequent day, the patient improved to an NIH stroke score of 1 for mild arm weakness, and CT perfusion was entirely symmetrical, with a small, previously completed infarct in the predicted core.

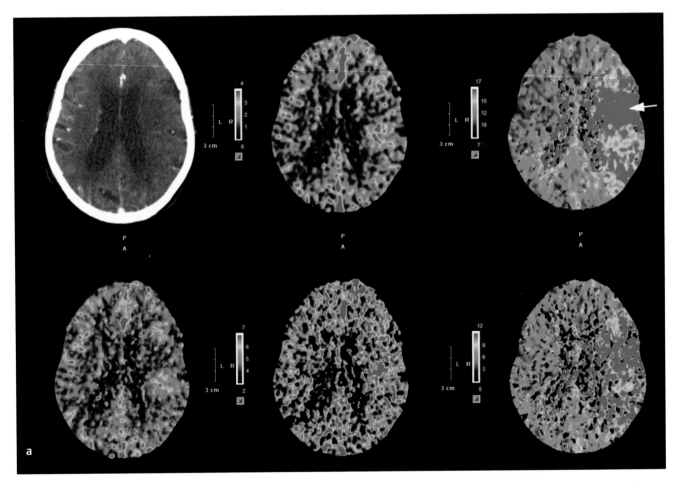

**Fig. 6.15** **(a)** A computed tomographic perfusion stroke study shows a left middle cerebral artery occlusion with hypoperfusion (*arrow*).

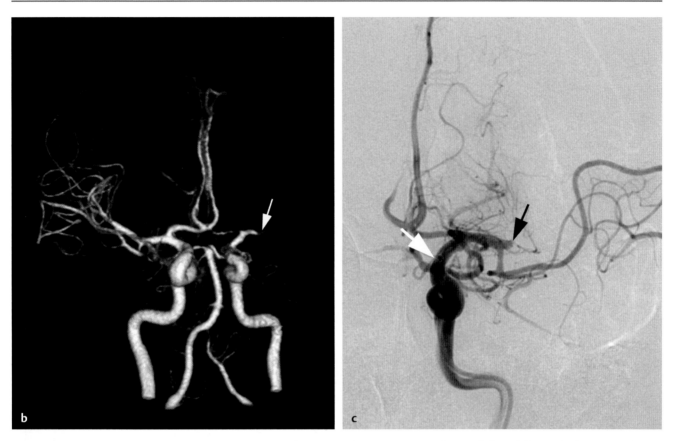

**Fig. 6.15** (*Continued*)   **(b)** Computed three-dimensional tomographic angiography shows a left middle cerebral artery occlusion (*arrow*). **(c)** A catheter (0.54 in, Penumbra, Inc., Alameda, CA) is placed in the supraclinoid left internal carotid artery (*left arrow*). The left middle cerebral artery is occluded at a large superior M2 segment (*right arrow*).

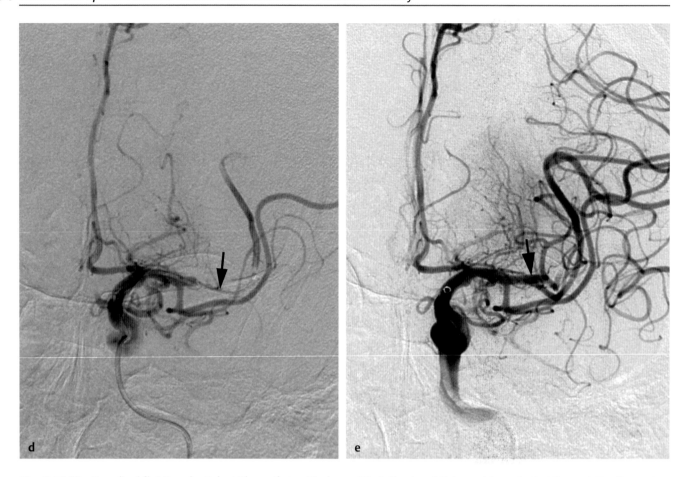

**Fig. 6.15** (*Continued*)   **(d)** A Prowler Select Plus catheter (Codman, West Chester, PA) (*arrow*) is navigated through the Penumbra and across the M2 segment of the middle cerebral artery stenosis in preparation for deploying the Solitaire (Covidien, Plymouth, MN). **(e)** Left internal carotid angiogram obtained after the Solitaire is deployed and suction is used through the Penumbra. The M2 segment is reopened (*arrow*) and full perfusion through the M1 segment as well.

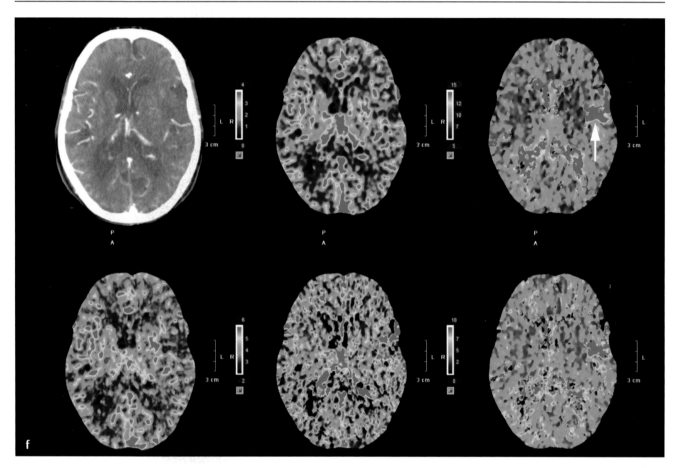

**Fig. 6.15** (*Continued*)    **(f)** The postintervention computed tomographic perfusion study. A small distal area of hypoperfusion in the left middle cerebral artery is evident (*arrow*).

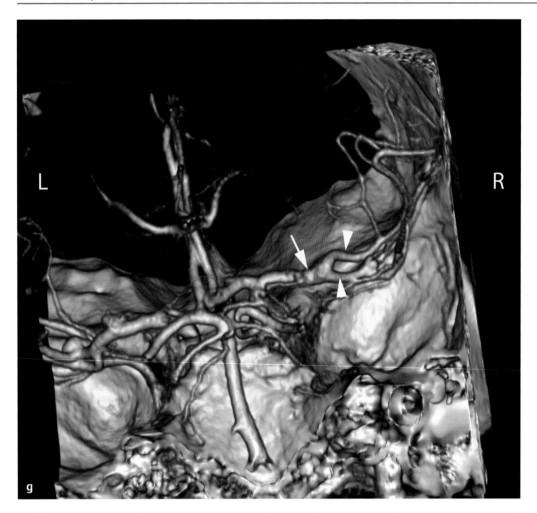

**Fig. 6.15** (*Continued*)   **(g)** Computed tomographic three-dimensional angiography shows patent M1 (*arrow*) and M2 segments (*arrowheads*).

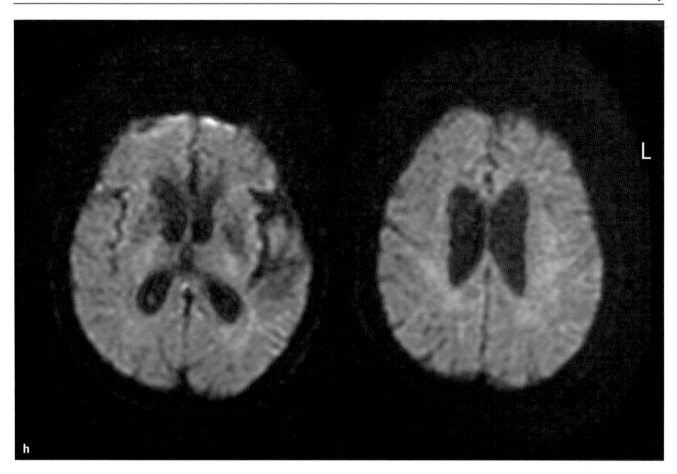

**Fig. 6.15** (*Continued*)  **(h)** Postintervention noncontrasted magnetic resonance imaging of the brain. No infarction of the brain is evident.

### 6.6.3 Case 3

A young teenager presented with a new-onset, generalized seizure. A computed tomographic scan suggested a possible right frontal vascular malformation. An angiogram confirmed the presence of an arteriovenous malformation (AVM) arising from branches of the superior trunk of the middle cerebral artery with venous drainage into the superficial veins. The patient was treated with anticonvulsants and brought for selective catheterization and embolization under conscious sedation. A microcatheter angiogram revealed the angioarchitecture of the AVM. Prior to embolization, the patient underwent a comprehensive neurological examination after instillation of amytal and lidocaine for a Wada test. Because there was no neurological deficit on examination, the AVM was embolized using a liquid embolic agent. This was performed for two arterial pedicles. Delayed angiography revealed complete obliteration of the AVM.

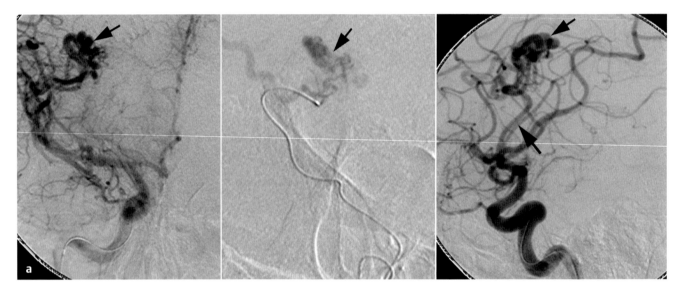

**Fig. 6.16**  **(a)** A right internal carotid angiogram shows an arteriovenous malformation (*upper arrows*) supplied by the distal segments of the right middle cerebral artery (*right lower arrow*).

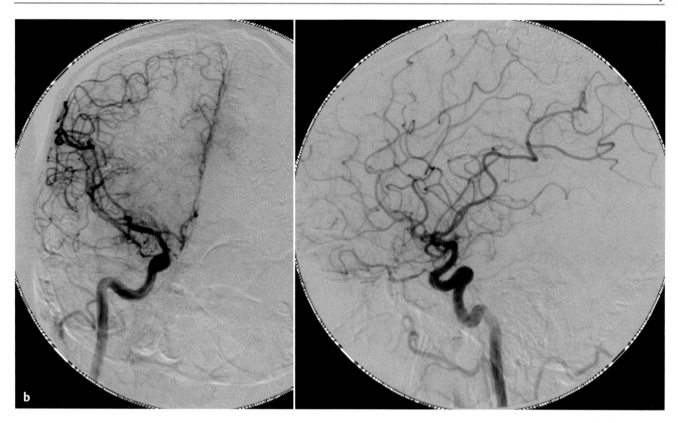

**Fig. 6.16** (*Continued*)  **(b)** Postendovascular embolization right carotid angiography shows complete obliteration of the arteriovenous malformation.

## Clinical Pearls

- Wide exposure of the Sylvian fissure provides an excellent demonstration of the entire proximal middle cerebral artery (MCA), including the M1, M2, and M3 segments. Therefore, craniotomy and clipping of typical wide-necked aneurysms at the MCA bifurcation is still the preferred interventional method. However, the lateral lenticulostriate vessels must not be compromised. These bifurcation aneurysms are very difficult to treat using standard endovascular techniques because of their wide-necked anatomy and concern for compromise of one or more M2 segments. Endovascular treatment frequently requires adjunctive techniques, such as the use of two stents, one in each M2, to create a Y stent construct followed by coiling. This technique significantly increases the risk of the endovascular procedure and is reserved for those unable to withstand craniotomy for clipping. Newer technologies, such as endosaccular flow diverters or bifurcation devices, may change the status quo.

- The distal M2 and proximal M3 branches serve as excellent, relatively superficial recipients of high-flow bypass using either vein or arterial interposition grafts.

### Anterior/Temporal

- This vessel is frequently key for providing collateral supply to preserve the penumbra along distal middle cerebral artery territories (especially temporal) during acute ischemic strokes from a distal M1 proximal M2 occlusions.

### Frontal

- These cortical M4 vessels serve as excellent recipients of the lower-flow superficial temporal artery direct arterial bypass.

- Aneurysms of the M1 segment and internal carotid (IC) artery bifurcation, however, have a higher surgical risk because of the myriad perforators, which can be hard to dissect free or visualize because of a deeper, more crowded field as compared to middle cerebral artery bifurcation aneurysms. Similarly, although flow diversion is an excellent option for proximal IC artery aneurysms, particularly those proximal to the posterior communicating artery, placement of flow diverters in the M1, especially more than one, risks compromise of the lenticulostriates and neurological sequelae. However, stent-assisted coiling remains an excellent option for many aneurysms in this location.

  M1 is the most common location of a large-vessel occlusion resulting in acute ischemic stroke. These occlusions are typically recalcitrant to intravenous thrombolytics, and new randomized trials suggest that they may be uniquely suitable for endovascular recanalization using stent retrievers and local thromboaspiration either separately or together.

# 7 Anterior Cerebral and Anterior Communicating Arteries

The anterior cerebral artery originates from bifurcation of the internal carotid artery just opposite the olfactory trigone. The segment that courses medially over the junction of the optic nerve with the chiasm to join the anterior communicating artery is designated as the A1. The A1 segment gives off perforators superiorly to the medial striate region and small perforators inferiorly to the chiasm and optic nerves. The anterior cerebral artery (A1), after joining the anterior communicating artery, continues superiorly and around the genu of the corpus callosum as the A2 segment. The orbital frontal and frontal polar branches originate from the A2 as it courses around the genu of the corpus callosum. The A2 subsequently divides into pericallosal and callosomarginal branches. The configuration of the anterior communicating artery and the distribution and configuration of the pericallosal artery and callosomarginal arteries vary widely. The anterior cerebral artery then distributes branches to the medial hemisphere, extending back and including the precuneus region. The distal and posterior portion of the pericallosal artery anastomoses through the microcirculation with the splenial artery from the posterior cerebral circulation.

## 7.1 A1 Segment

The diameter of the A1 segment varies widely. When the segment on one side is hypoplastic, the opposite is usually significantly enlarged. Complete absence of the A1 segment on one side is rare. The A1 segment can actually penetrate the optic nerve or chiasm, but this was not found in the senior author's specimens. The A1 segment may be fenestrated.

## 7.2 Heubner's Artery

Heubner's artery originates in the region at the junction of the A1, the anterior communicating artery, and the A2 segments. It can originate in the midportion of the A1 segment. The artery courses laterally, frequently hidden by the A1 segment, and terminates just medial to the lateral striate branches of the middle cerebral artery. Heubner's artery may be double on either one or both sides. However, its absence was not found by the author and is probably very rare.

## 7.3 Anterior Communicating Artery

The anterior communicating artery joins the two A1 segments in the midline and gives origin to the two A2 segments. This configuration is extremely variable, and the complete absence of an anterior communicating artery is rare. The anterior communicating artery may be represented by multiple bridges and fenestrations. It gives rise to perforators that extend posteriorly to the hypothalamic region.

## 7.4 A2 Segment

The A2 segment originates after the A1 joins the anterior communicating artery. The A2 segments on either side usually have approximately equal diameter, but their branches may be variable. However, the orbital frontal and frontal polar branches are very consistent, and the orbital frontal branch usually originates about 5 mm to 1 cm after the origin of the A2 from the anterior communicating artery. At times, there may be a single A2 segment or a triple A2 segment.

## 7.5 Pericallosal Artery

The pericallosal artery is the direct continuation of the A2 segment. It extends posteriorly, and at the splenium of the corpus callosum anastomoses with the microcirculation of the splenial artery of the posterior cerebral artery. It also terminates in branches going to the precuneus. However, the branching and relationship with the callosomarginal artery are widely variable. At times, the pericallosal artery has the configuration of the main artery of the medial hemisphere, giving off branches in a spokelike fashion to supply the gyri of the medial hemisphere. On occasion, there may be crossover links between the pericallosal arteries of each side.

## 7.6 Callosomarginal Artery

The callosomarginal artery is also a continuation of the A2 segment. It passes superiorly to the cingulate gyrus and supplies the anterior frontal lobe and the paracentral lobule superiorly. The configuration and branches of the callosomarginal artery are also variable, but crossover between the two callosomarginal arteries is much less common than is found with the pericallosal artery.

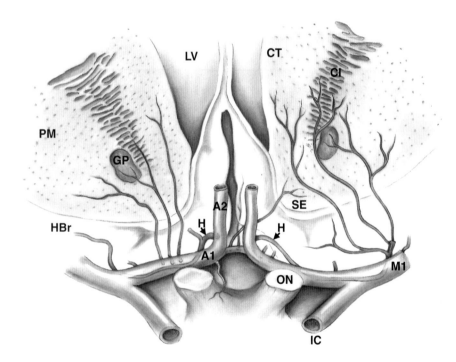

**Fig. 7.1**   A coronal section of the cerebral hemispheres at the level of the beginning of the globus pallidus. A1 and the anterior communicating artery perforator patterns are shown.

A1   anterior cerebral artery
A2   anterior cerebral artery
CI   internal capsule
CT   caudate nucleus
GP   globus pallidus
H   Heubner's artery
HBr   Heubner's artery to frontal lobe
LV   lateral ventricle
M1   middle cerebral artery
ON   optic nerve
PM   putamen
SE   septal area
IC   internal carotid artery

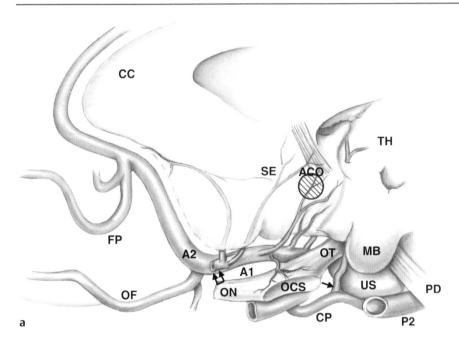

**Fig. 7.2** **(a)** A sagittal section through the corpus callosum at the level of the optic chiasm. A medial view of the right hemisphere.

A1   anterior cerebral artery
A2   anterior cerebral artery
ACO  anterior commissure
CC   corpus callosum
CP   posterior communicating artery
FP   frontopolar artery
MB   mammillary body
OCS  optic chiasm
ON   optic nerve
OF   orbitofrontal artery
OT   optic tract
PD   peduncle
P2   posterior cerebral artery
SE   septal area
TH   thalamus
US   uncus
→    premammillary artery
⇉    anterior communicating artery

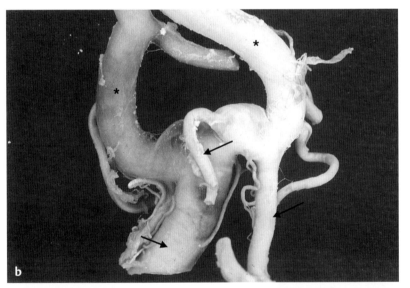

**Fig. 7.2** **(b,c)** Anterior communicating artery region illustrating "third A2," which becomes the subcallosal artery. **(b)** Posterior view. Subcallosal artery (*right upper arrow*); A1s (*right lower arrow, left lower arrow*); A2s (*\**). **(c)** Anterior view. Orbito-frontal artery (*white arrow*); A1s (*right lower arrow, left lower arrow*); A2s (*\**).

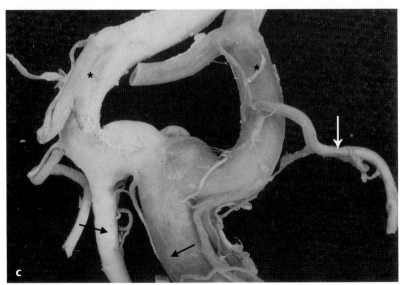

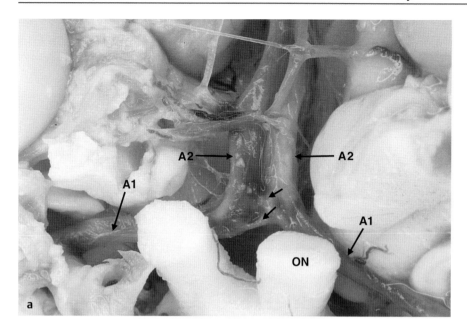

**Fig. 7.3** **(a)** A double anterior communicating artery (*arrows*) with symmetrical A1 and A2 segments.

A1  anterior cerebral artery
A2  anterior cerebral artery
ON  optic nerve

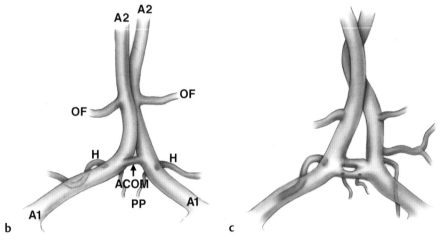

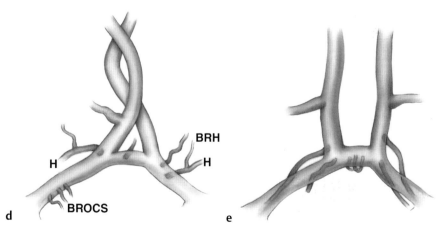

**Fig. 7.3** **(b–e)** Variations of the configuration of the anterior communicating artery region. All perforators are not shown in each figure. See **Fig. 7.4** regarding Heubner's artery. **(r)**, **(s)**, and **(t)** show incidental aneurysms found on postmortem.

A1      anterior cerebral artery
A2      anterior cerebral artery
ACOM    anterior communicating artery
BROCS   br. to optic chiasm
BRH     br. to frontal lobe
H       Heubner's artery
OF      orbital-frontal artery
PP      perforators

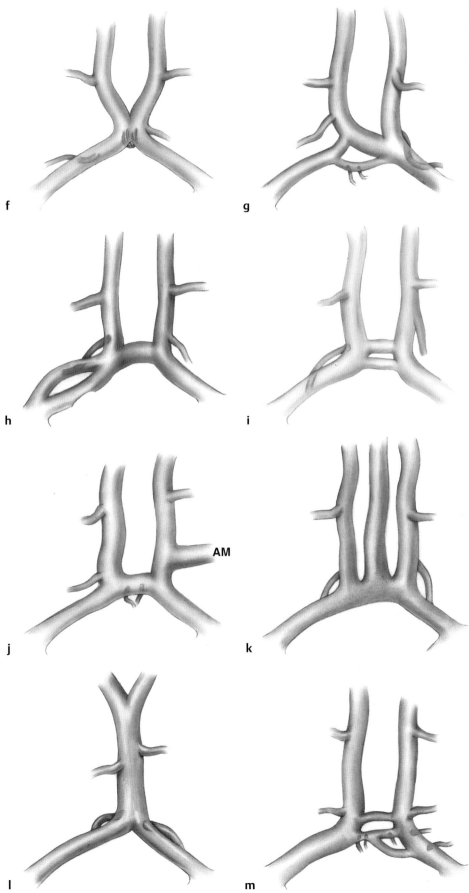

**Fig. 7.3 (f–m)** Variations of the configuration of the anterior communicating artery region.

AM   accessory middle cerebral artery in **Fig. 7.3j**

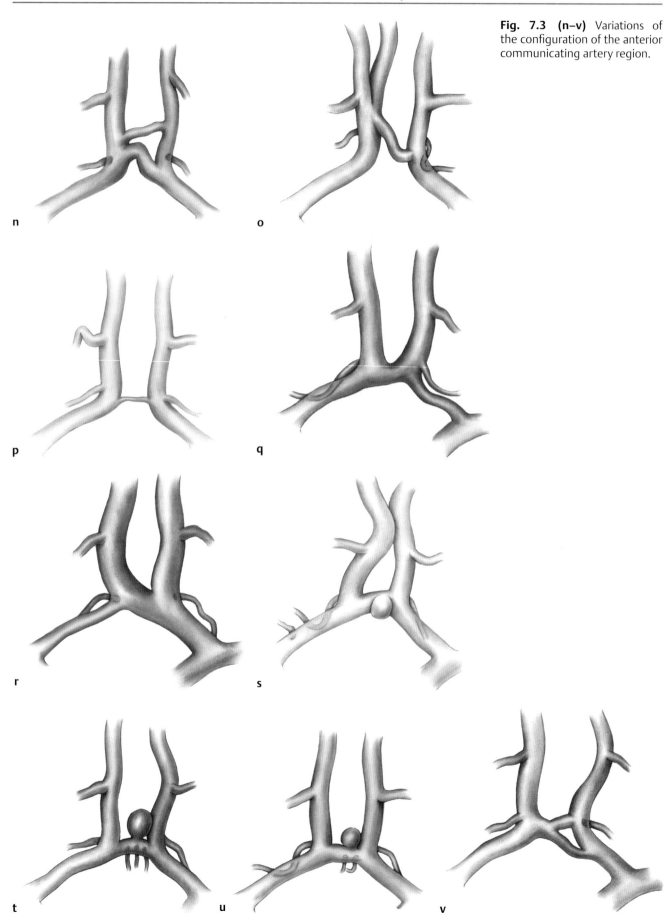

**Fig. 7.3 (n–v)** Variations of the configuration of the anterior communicating artery region.

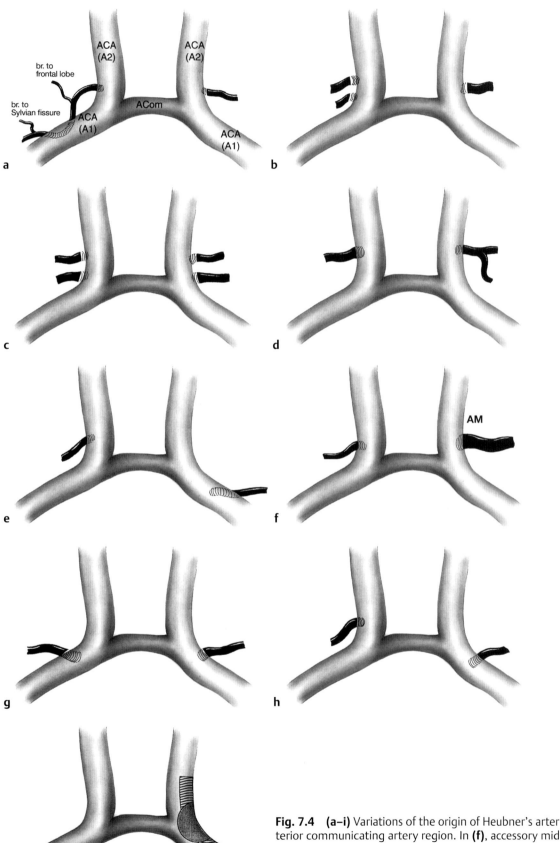

**Fig. 7.4** **(a–i)** Variations of the origin of Heubner's artery (*black*) at the anterior communicating artery region. In **(f)**, accessory middle cerebral artery (AM) goes to Sylvian fissure.

ACA    anterior cerebral artery
ACom   anterior communicating artery

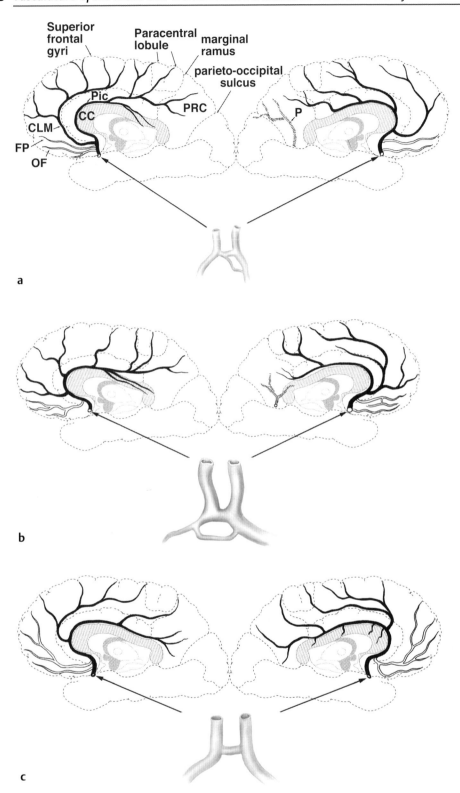

**Fig. 7.5** The configurations of the distal anterior cerebral arteries. Medial view of matching hemispheres. The anterior communicating artery of each brain is shown. Note that in **(j)**, the anterior communicating artery was damaged and is not shown. **(a,b)** Terminal attenuation of the pericallosal artery (see **Fig. 7.6b**). **(c)** Prominence of the orbital frontal and frontal polar distribution. **(e)** A rare small crossover between the callosomarginal arteries. **(e,f)** Prominence of the posterior cerebral circulation to the precuneus region; **(e)** also shows absence of the pericallosal artery in the left hemisphere. **(g–n)** Crossover configurations of the pericallosal artery. Note the variability of the branches of the pericallosal and callosomarginal arteries to the superior frontal gyrus, paracentral lobule, and precuneus **(a–n)**.

CC      corpus callosum
CLM    callosomarginal artery
FP       frontopolar artery
OF       orbitofrontal artery
P         posterior cerebral artery
Pic      pericallosal artery
PRC     precuneus

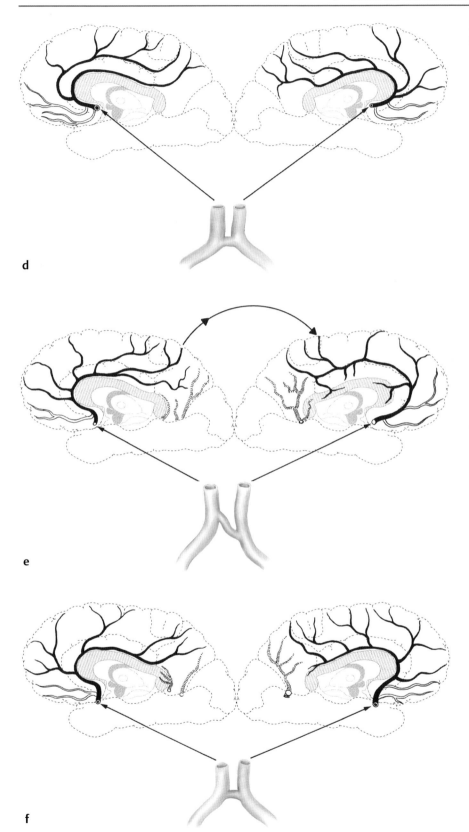

**Fig. 7.5 (d–f)** The configurations of the distal anterior cerebral arteries.

d

e

f

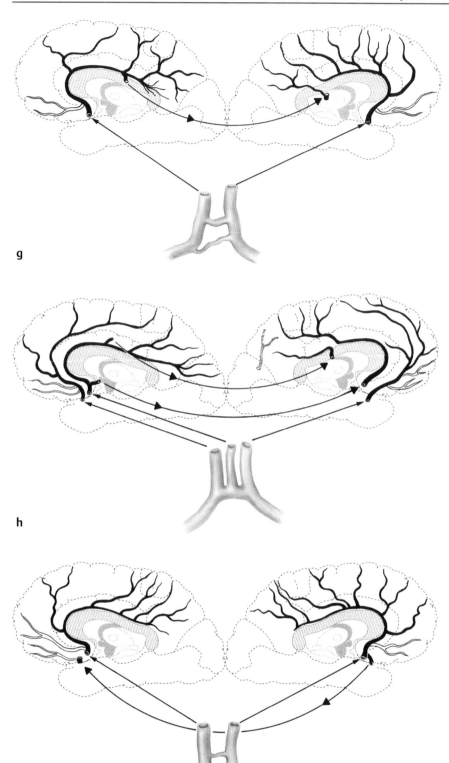

**Fig. 7.5 (g–i)** The configurations of the distal anterior cerebral arteries.

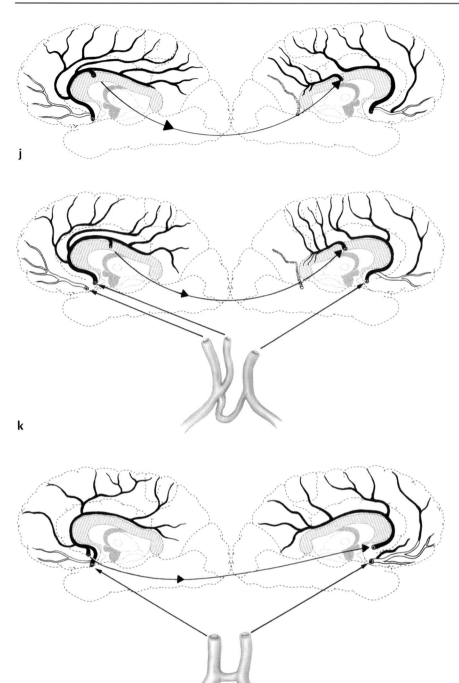

**Fig. 7.5 (j–l)** The configurations of the distal anterior cerebral arteries.

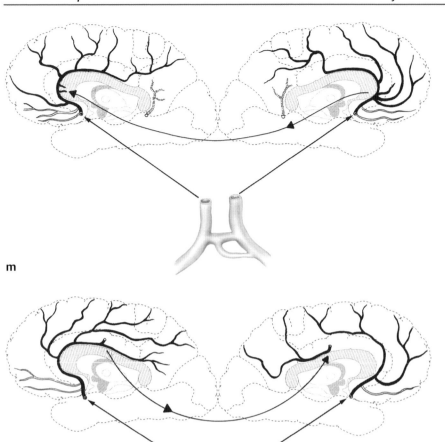

m

n

**Fig. 7.5 (m,n)** The configurations of the distal anterior cerebral arteries.

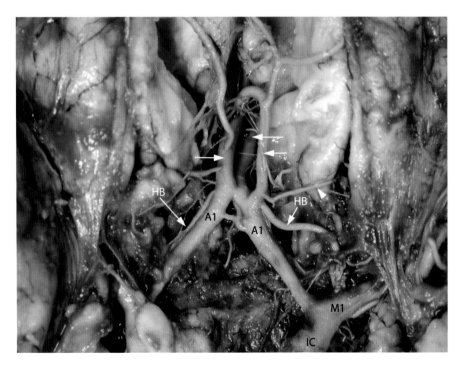

**Fig. 7.6** Ventral view of anterior circle of Willis. There are three A2s (*upper 3 arrows*) from the anterior communicating artery.

HB   Heubner's artery
A1   proximal anterior cerebral artery
M1   middle cerebral artery
IC   internal carotid artery
Arrowhead   orbito-frontal branch

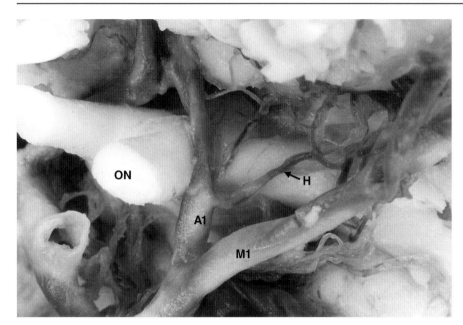

**Fig. 7.7** Heubner's artery originating from the midportion of A1.

A1 anterior cerebral artery
H Heubner's artery
M1 middle cerebral artery
ON optic nerve

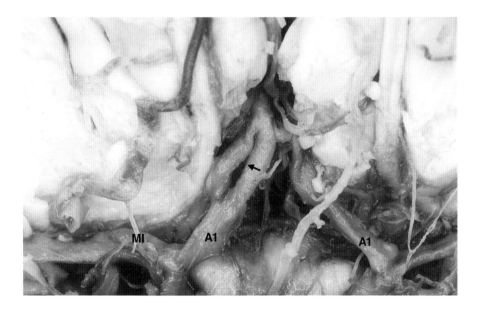

**Fig. 7.8** A frontal view of the supra-chiasmatic region. Fenestration (*arrow*) in the right A1 segment (A1) prior to union at the anterior communicating artery region.

A1 anterior cerebral artery
M1 middle cerebral artery

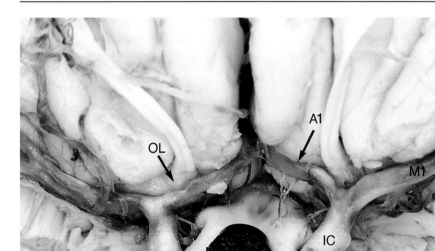

**Fig. 7.9** Frontal view of the suprachiasmatic region. The bifurcation of the carotid arteries opposite the olfactory trigone, and the medial course of the A1 segments is shown. The anterior communicating artery is partially hidden by the gyrus rectus.

A1    anterior cerebral artery
IC    internal carotid artery
M1    middle cerebral artery
OL    olfactory trigone

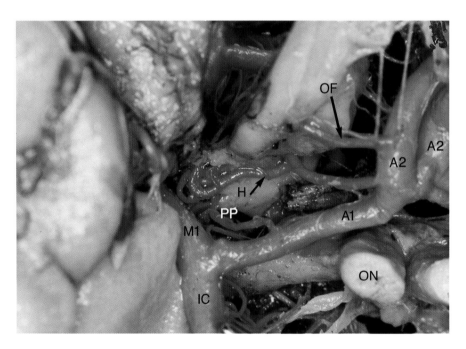

**Fig. 7.10** A1–A2 junction and the origin of A1 from the internal carotid (IC) artery. Heubner's artery (H) can be seen passing above and behind the A1 segment, terminating just medial to the lenticulostriate arteries.

A1    anterior cerebral artery
A2    anterior cerebral artery
M1    middle cerebral artery
OF    orbito-frontal branch
ON    optic nerve
PP    perforator

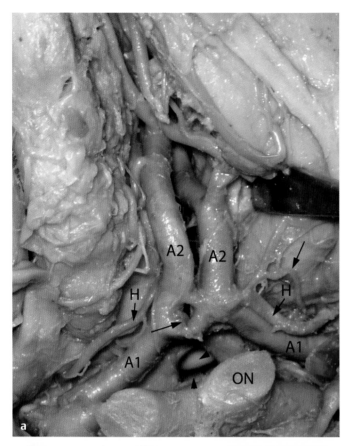

**Fig. 7.11** **(a)** Frontal view of anterior cerebral and anterior communicating artery complex. Heubner's artery (H) on left of the figure arises from A2 and, on right, the larger one arises from the junction of A1 and A2 and gives a branch (*single arrow on right*) to the frontal lobe. The anterior communicating artery (*left arrow*) is double with a fenestration (see **Figs. 7.3i** and **7.3v**). Optic nerve (ON), opened lamina terminalis (*lower arrowhead*) with view of anterior commissure (*upper arrowhead*) crossing third ventricle.

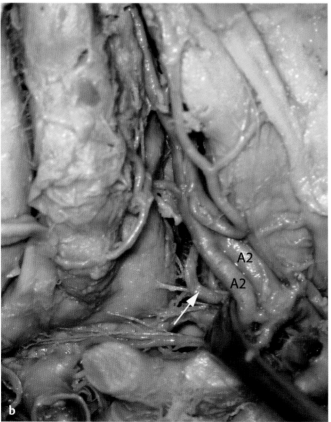

**Fig. 7.11** **(b)** Same specimen as **Fig. 7.11a**. Retracting the anterior communicating artery complex reveals a large perforator (*arrow*) originating from the anterior communicating artery coursing posteriorly toward the preseptal area.

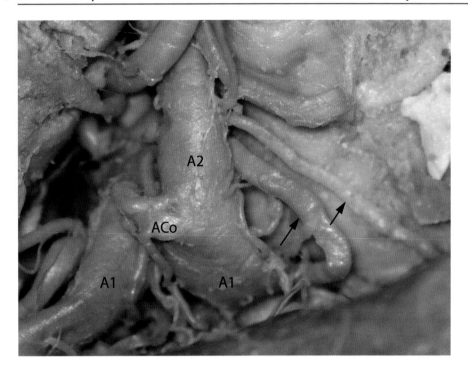

**Fig. 7.12** Frontal view of anterior communicating complex. Two Heubner's arteries (*two arrows*) arise from A2.

A1    anterior cerebral artery
ACO  anterior communicating artery
      (see **Fig. 7.4b**)

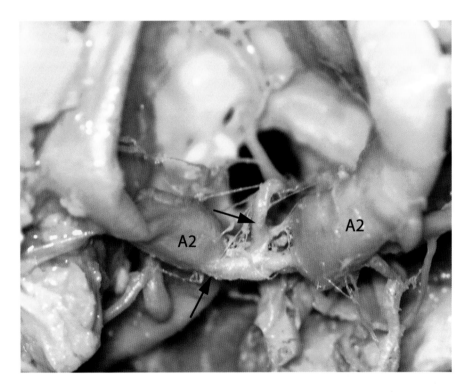

**Fig. 7.13** Precallosal artery (*upper arrow*) arising from the back of anterior communicating artery (*lower arrow*).

A2  anterior cerebral artery

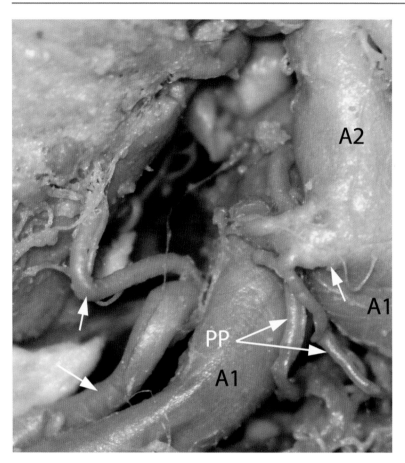

**Fig. 7.14** Heubner's artery (*left lower arrow*) gives off a branch to the frontal lobe (*left upper arrow*).

A1   proximal anterior cerebral arteries; A2 is seen on right
PP   perforators

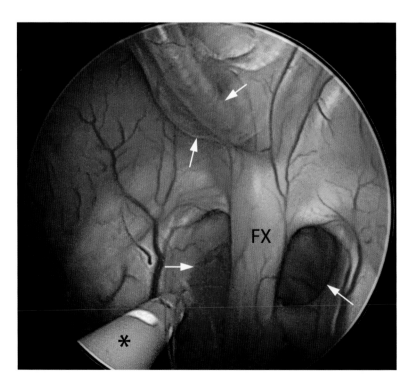

**Fig. 7.15** Endoscopic view into right lateral ventricle with septum pellucidum absent. Unusual course of the two A2s (*upper two arrows*) as they traverse the ventricular system before going over the corpus callosum (*not visible*).

FX   fornix
Right lower arrow   right foramen of Monro
Left lower arrow     left foramen of Monro
*      ventricular catheter

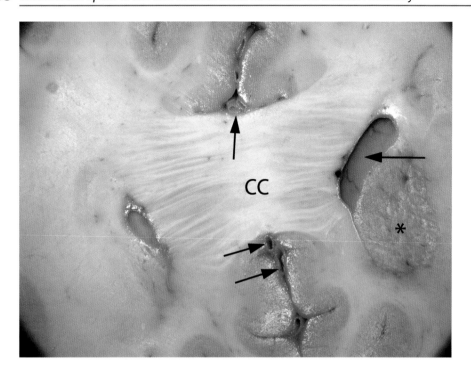

**Fig. 7.16** Coronal section through the rostrum of the corpus callosum (CC). The two pericallosal arteries above the corpus callosum (*upper arrow*) and below the corpus callosum (*lower arrows*).

\* head of the caudate nucleus
Right arrow   frontal horn

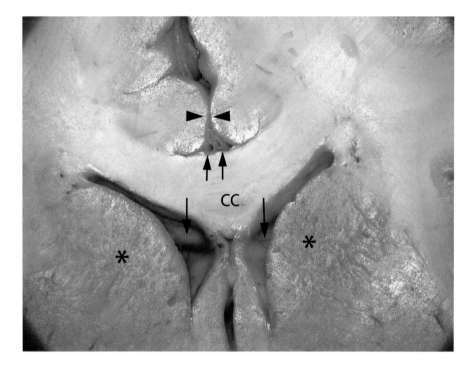

**Fig. 7.17** Coronal section 2 cm posterior to **Fig. 7.16**. The cingulate gyri (*opposite arrowheads*) oppose each other, covering the pericallosal arteries (*upper arrows*) lying on the corpus callosum below (CC).

\* caudate nucleus
Lower arrows   lateral ventricles

## 7.7 Cinical Cases

### 7.7.1 Case 1

A middle-aged woman was found by her family to be obtunded and brought to the hospital. Computed tomography (CT) showed diffuse subarachnoid hemorrhage with a focal interhemispheric clot and a large left intracerebral hematoma. An emergent ventriculostomy was placed, and the patient was brought to the angiography suite. The angiogram revealed a large, irregularly shaped anterior communicating artery (ACom) aneurysm filling primarily from the left anterior cerebral artery (ACA). The aneurysm was catheterized and primarily coiled. The following day, because of increasing intracranial pressures and a large intracerebral hematoma, the patient was taken to the operating room. A small craniotomy was performed through the left eyebrow, and the clot was evacuated using endoscopic and ultrasound assistance. The patient had a protracted hospital course but at 6 months was independent and at home.

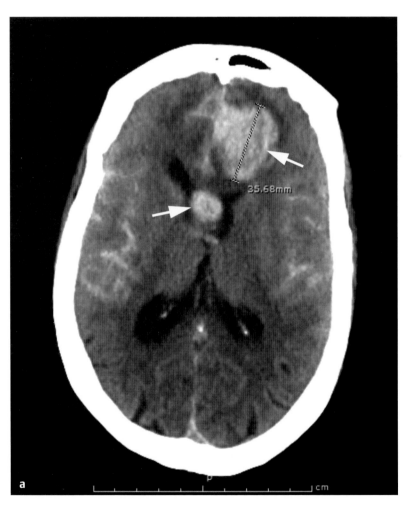

**Fig. 7.18   (a)** Noncontrasted computed tomography of the head shows a ruptured anterior communicating artery aneurysm with a left frontal hematoma (*upper arrow*). There is blood in the lateral ventricles (*lower arrow*).

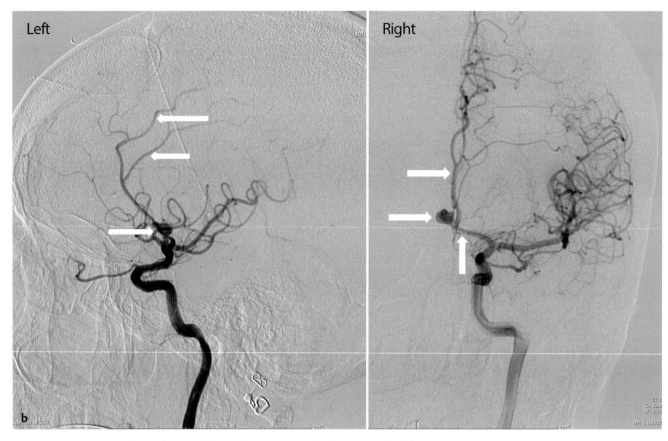

**Fig. 7.18** (*Continued*) **(b)** Left internal carotid angiogram. The figure on the left (lateral view) shows the callosal marginal artery (*upper arrow*), pericallosal artery (*middle arrow*), and aneurysm (*lower arrow*). The figure on the right (anteroposterior view) shows the left anterior cerebral artery (A2) (*upper arrow*), left anterior cerebral artery (A1) (*lower arrow*), and anterior communicating artery aneurysm (*middle arrow*).

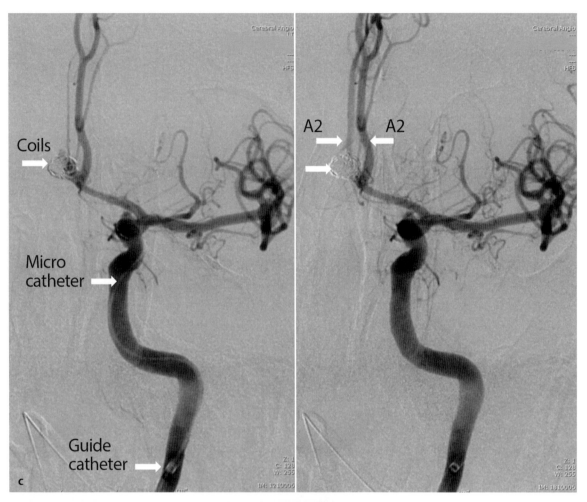

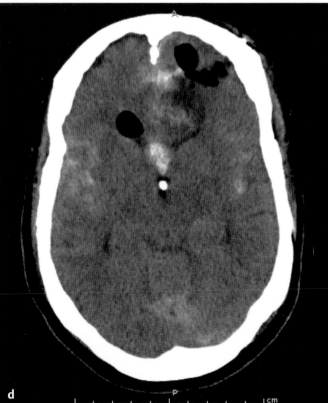

**Fig. 7.18** (*Continued*)    **(c)** Coil embolization of the aneurysm. The figure on the left shows coiling in progress. In the figure on the right, coiling is completed (*arrow*). Both A2s of the anterior cerebral arteries are filling distal to the coiled aneurysm. **(d)** Noncontrasted computed tomographic head scan on day 1 after evacuation of the left frontal hematoma postcoiling.

## 7.7.2 Case 2

A middle-aged woman with a chronic history of headaches that were becoming worse, with early cognitive decline, presented with a concern for an arteriovenous malformation seen on computed tomography (CT). Angiography revealed a rare galenic malformation variant with a direct perical-losal fistula into a dilated variceal falcine vein and additional smaller direct fistulae from distal posterior cerebral branches around the splenium of the corpus callosum. Under general anesthesia and hypotension, the flow was occluded through the pericallosal artery using a balloon, and the varix was occluded using a combination of coils and liquid embolic. At the completion of the procedure there was slow, delayed filling from a few posterior cerebral branches distal to the occluded varix. The patient was maintained under hypotension for an additional 48 hours. Repeat angiography prior to discharge at 7 days and again at 6 months revealed complete occlusion of the fistula. The patient was able to return from recent transfer to an assisted living facility back to independent living.

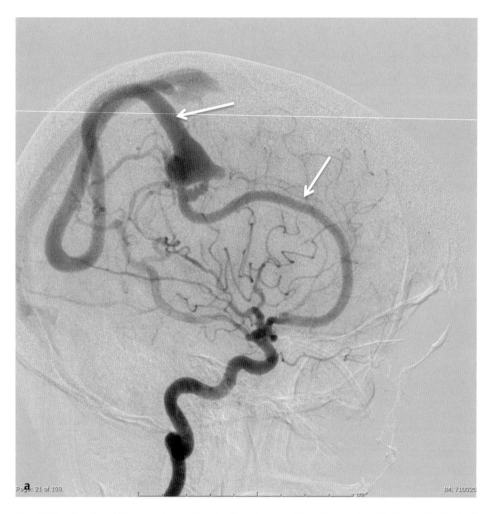

**Fig. 7.19** **(a)** A right internal carotid injection shows a high-flow vein of Galen variant arteriovenous fistula. A superficial draining vein (*upper arrow*) and pericallosal artery (*lower arrow*) are visible.

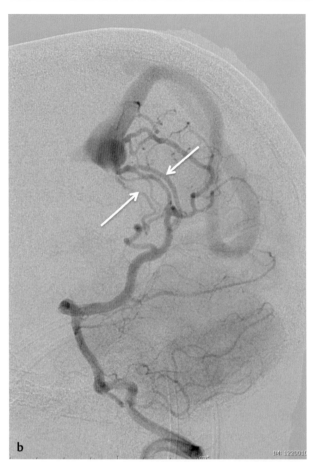

**Fig. 7.19** (*Continued*)   **(b)** A left lateral vertebral angiogram shows the left posterior medial choroidal artery (*left arrow*) and left lateral posterior choroidal artery (*right arrow*). **(c)** Contribution to the fistula by the right anterior cerebral artery (*left arrow*) and the right posterior cerebral artery (*right arrow*).

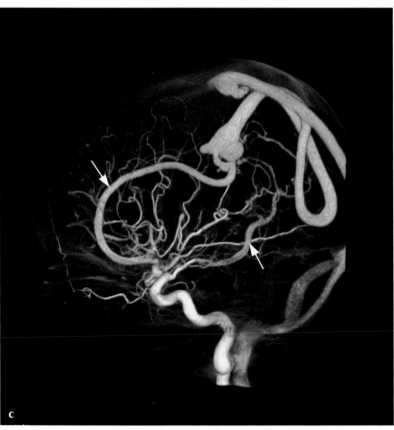

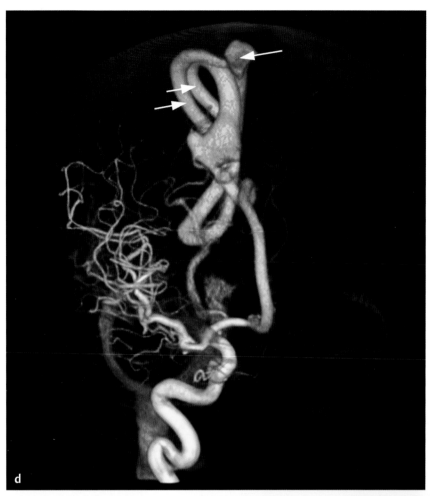

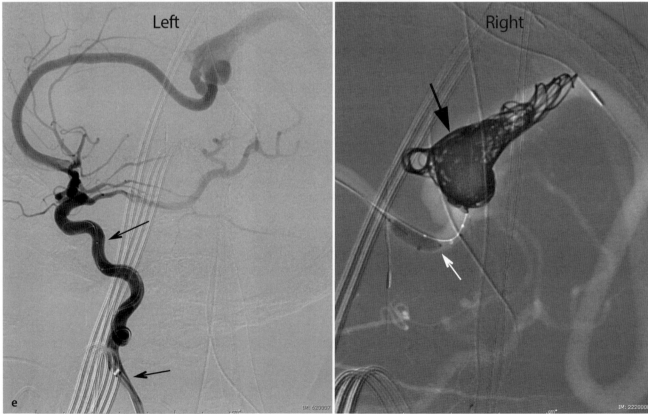

**Fig. 7.19** (*Continued*) **(d)** The fistula drains into tortuous cortical veins (*left arrows*) and then into the superior sagittal sinus (*right arrow*). **(e)** Right internal carotid angiogram. On the left is a microcatheter (*arrows*) with a Scepter C balloon (4 × 10 mm, Microvention, Inc., Tustin, CA), and on the right a Scepter C balloon (*lower arrow*) and coils in the fistula (*upper arrow*).

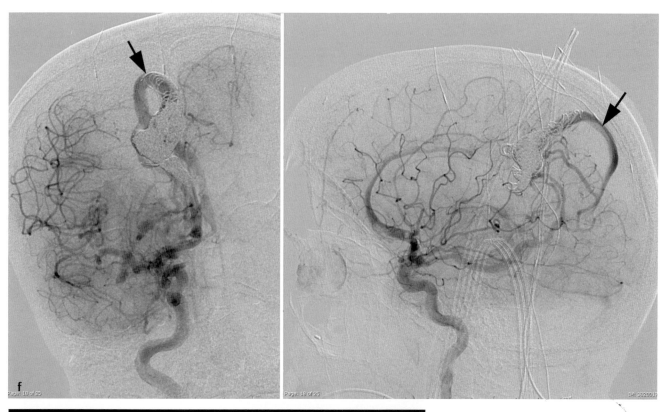

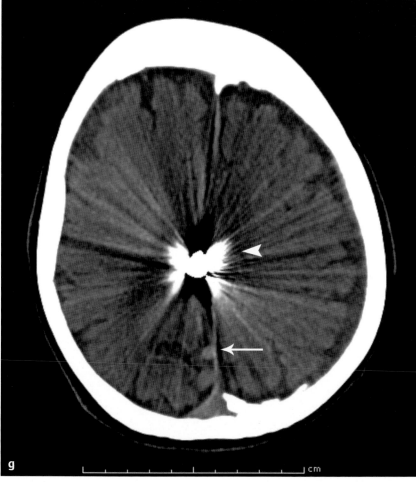

**Fig. 7.19** (*Continued*) **(f)** Right internal carotid angiogram. The anterior cerebral artery contribution is occluded, but the fistula is still open. There is slower filling and contrast stasis in the draining vein (*arrows*). **(g)** Metal artifact of coil mass (*arrowhead*) without evidence of hemorrhage, with hyperintensity of the vein with slowed flow (*arrow*).

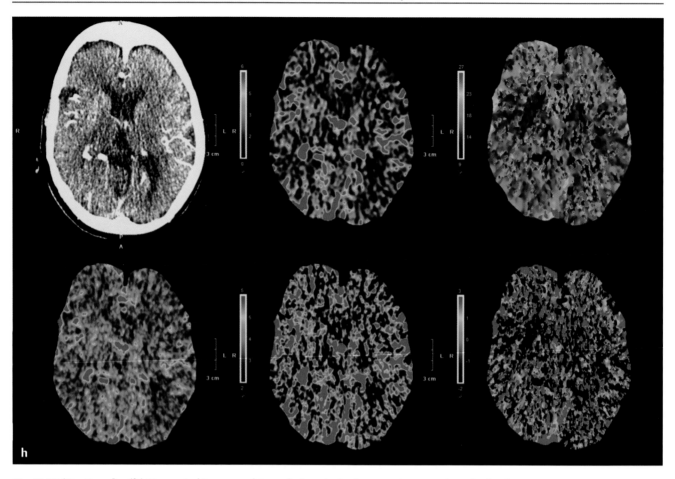

**Fig. 7.19** (*Continued*)  **(h)** Computed tomographic perfusion study shows no increased cerebral volume.

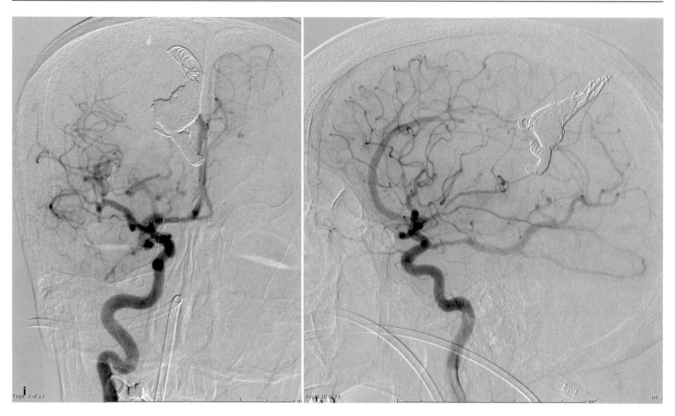

**Fig. 7.19** (*Continued*)   **(i)** Delayed phase in a right internal carotid angiogram. There is no filling of the fistula.

### 7.7.3 Case 3

A middle-aged woman presented with incidental discovery of multiple aneurysms found during a chronic headache workup. On angiography she was noted to have a hypoplastic right A1 and a dominant left A1 segment supplying both A2 segments, as well as an anterior communicating artery (ACom) aneurysm arising at the junction of the left A1 and A2. Although initially planned to be treated with a stent from the right A2 to the left A1 across the ACom aneurysm, she was noted to fill the right A2 through multiple small ACom channels, and the aneurysm was asymmetric to the left A2–A1 junction. She was also noted to have a small left superior hypophyseal artery aneurysm. She was brought to the angiography suite after ensuring she was therapeutic on dual antiplatelet agents. A microcatheter was placed into the distal left A2 and a braided microstent was positioned across the ACom aneurysm from the left A2 to the left A1. A second microcatheter, which had previously been jailed into the aneurysm, was used to coil the aneurysm. At 6 months there was complete occlusion of the aneurysm and the patient remained asymptomatic.

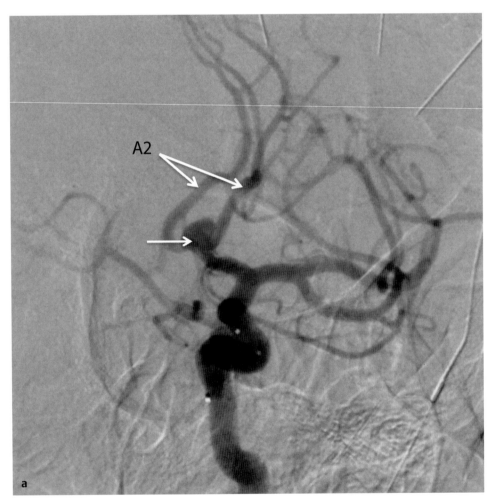

**Fig. 7.20** **(a)** A left internal carotid angiogram shows an anterior communicating artery aneurysm (*lower arrow*). Anterior cerebral arteries (A2) are seen on either side (*upper arrows*).

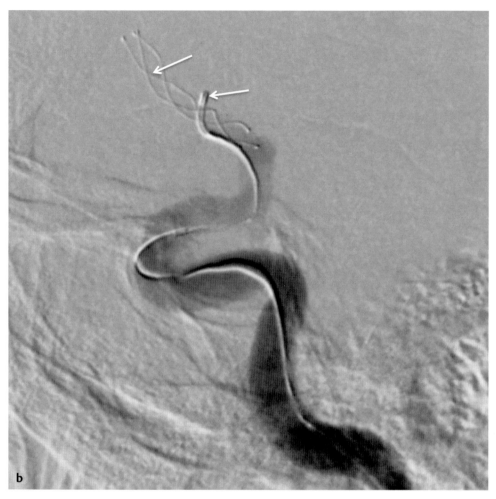

**Fig. 7.20** (*Continued*)    **(b)** Microcatheter in place for coiling (*arrows*).

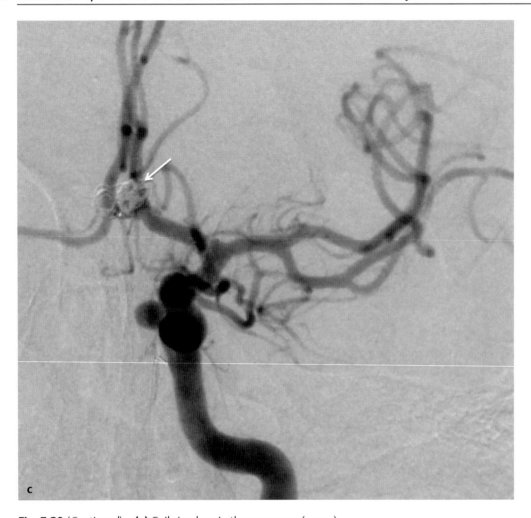

**Fig. 7.20** (*Continued*)   **(c)** Coils in place in the aneurysm (*arrow*).

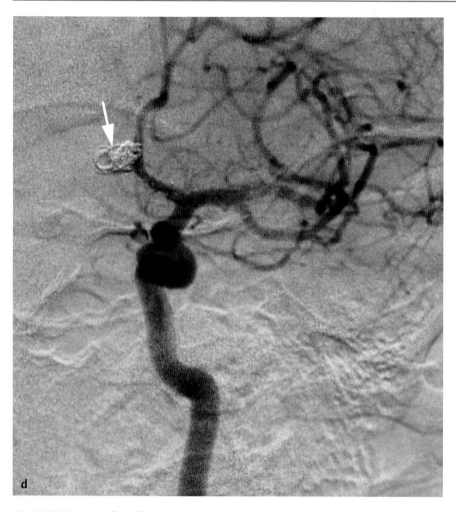

**Fig. 7.20** (*Continued*)   **(d)** The aneurysm (*arrow*) is completely obliterated by coils.

## Clinical Pearls

- The A2 subsequently divides. The A1 segment can actually penetrate the optic nerve or chiasm. It rarely originates directly from the clinoidal segment of the carotid artery and passes below the optic nerve to the anterior communicating artery, but this was not found in the senior author's specimens. The A1 segment may be fenestrated.

- During craniotomy for clipping anterior communicating artery (ACom) aneurysms, the A1 can reliably be exposed directly above the optic nerve. Unless the aneurysm is pointing down and forward and the ACom is low lying, a small area of gyrus rectus resection is frequently required to adequately expose the proximal A2 segments to complete dissection of the H complex consisting of the two A1s, A2s, and ACom arteries.

  During endovascular catheterization of the A1 segment, ideally the microcatheter should be placed with the distal tip in the clinoidal segment at or just proximal to the origin of the ophthalmic artery, and the microwire is used to select the A1 artery. If the microcatheter is placed distal or proximal to the clinoidal segment, then the wire typically tends to find the M1 segment

### Heubner's Artery

- Heubner's artery supplies the medial-basal ganglia, including most prominently the head of the caudate nucleus.

- Excessive manipulation or postprocedure spasm of Heubner's artery may result in infarction of the head of the caudate after clipping of ACom aneurysms. It presents with mild somnolesence and mild hemiparesis, which rapidly resolve over the subsequent few days, with a telltale sign on head computed tomography.

### Anterior Communicating Artery and Optic Chiasm

- The ACom is frequently fenestrated and highly subject to flow-related misinterpretation of angiographic anatomy. To best visualize the precise anatomy, either a combined bilateral carotid angiogram or contralateral carotid artery compression angiogram is required.

  ACom aneurysms are among the most common ruptured aneurysms and tend to rupture at smaller sizes. This may be related to the variable anatomy in this region and the multiple fenestrations affecting wall-shear stress. Although anterior-inferior pointing aneurysms are safely treated through craniotomy, posterior-superior directed aneurysms pose additional risks given the need for greater retraction and resection to

visualize the H complex anatomy, as well as a greater presence of the hypothalamic perforators around the aneurysm neck.

Endovascular treatment is hampered by the angle of the A1 segment off the carotid artery, which increases difficulty with access and stability. Frequent fenestrations can also complicate desired stent deployment, especially if the plan is to go across the ACom from one A1 to the contralateral A2.

### A2 Segment

- Aneurysms of the A2 segment frequently tend to be fusiform, likely related to the proximity of the rigid falx cerebri, and therefore etiologically related to an underlying dissection. They are best treated endovascularly, or, when saccular, through an interhemispheric approach because of the extensive retraction required for visualization through a pterional craniotomy.

### Pericallosal Artery

- The pericallosal artery is the direct continuation of the A2 segment, typically named pericallosal as it emerges around the superior edge of the genu of the corpus callosum. It extends posteriorly and, at the splenium of the corpus callosum, anastomoses with the microcirculation of the splenial artery, a branch of the posterior cerebral artery. It also terminates in branches going to the precuneus. However, the branching and relationship with the callosomarginal artery are quite variable. At times, the pericallosal artery has the configuration of the main artery of the medial hemisphere, giving off branches in a spokelike fashion to supply the gyri of the medial hemisphere. On occasion, there may be crossover links between the pericallosal arteries of each side.

- In cases where a bypass is required, such as during repair of a giant ACom or A2 aneurysm, the presence of the two pericallosal arteries in close proximity over the corpus callosum provides an ideal location for a side-to-side bypass between the two A3 arteries.

  During clipping of pericallosal aneurysms, it is advantageous to have frameless stereotactic navigation available to optimize the approach angle, minimize dissection, and reduce operative struggle in locating the aneurysm, which may be hidden by interdigitated cingulate gyri through a deficient falx cerebri.

  Frequently, in cases of moyamoya disease, the splenial artery anastomosis is critical in preventing anterior cerebral ischemia.

# 8 Basilar Bifurcation and Posterior Cerebral Arteries

## 8.1 Course and Segments of the Posterior Cerebral Artery

The posterior cerebral arteries originate from the terminal bifurcation of the basilar artery on the ventral surface of the superior pons. The bifurcation of the basilar artery is at an acute angle so that the first portion of each posterior cerebral artery extends a few millimeters superiorly before turning laterally around the peduncle. The initial portion of the posterior cerebral artery is joined by the posterior communicating artery. That portion of the posterior cerebral artery between the basilar bifurcation and joining the posterior communicating artery is designated as P1. Arising from the P1 segment are perforators coursing into the interpeduncular fossa and the long circumferential quadrigeminal artery. The junction of the posterior communicating artery and P1 segment is frequently medial to the emergence of the third nerve, but on occasion is lateral to the origin of the third nerve.

Each posterior cerebral artery courses laterally and then turns superiorly around the peduncle. The posterior cerebral artery segment distal to the junction with the posterior communicating artery is designated P2. The very proximal P2 segment gives rise to the posterior medial choroidal artery. The P2 segment also supplies small perforators to the peduncle. The P2 contributes larger branches to the anterior and middle portions of the temporal lobe, as well as the uncus. The quadrigeminal artery and the posterior medial choroidal artery, as long circumferential vessels, are medial to the P2, as all three arteries course around the peduncles. The quadrigeminal and posterior medial choroidal arteries are covered in an arachnoid sheath and can adhere closely to the peduncle as they proceed posteriorly. The P2 is frequently buried deep in the choroidal fissure as it courses around the midbrain and may be covered with a tough arachnoid membrane. As the P2 arrives opposite the lateral and medial geniculate bodies at the base of the quadrigeminal cistern, it gives off a series of perforators, called the thalamogeniculate perforators, that enter the substance of the midbrain between the medial and lateral geniculate bodies. In the quadrigeminal cistern, the P2 can become coiled and looped and extends just opposite and inferior to the splenium of the corpus callosum to bury itself in the anterior aspect of the calcarine fissure. The P2 usually has its major bifurcation within the calcarine fissure, giving rise to the parietal occipital artery (P3) segments. At this major bifurcation, one branch becomes the P3, coursing posteriorly and entering the parietal occipital sulcus and ascending between the cuneus and precuneus. The other major branch of the P3 is a temporal occipital branch that gives rise to the calcarine artery, which may be double or triple. The other major branches are the occipital or posterior temporal branches and, on occasion, the lingual artery. At times, the anterior and middle temporal branches of the P2 have been referred to as the parahippocampal arteries, which produce a rakelike appearance on the anteroposterior angiogram. The entrance of the P2 into the quadrigeminal cistern is the point of transition from P2 to P3.

Just as the P2 enters the anterior calcarine sulcus, it gives off the splenial artery, which runs superior to the splenium of the corpus callosum and proceeds anteriorly to anastomose with the small terminal branches of the pericallosal artery of the anterior cerebral artery.

The posterior lateral choroidal arteries may be multiple and arise from the P2 segment or from branches of the P3 segments to supply the choroid plexus of the lateral ventricles at the trigone.

## 8.2 Posterior Thalamoperforators

The perforators arising from the region of the basilar bifurcation and P1 segments of the P2 are the posterior thalamoperforating arteries (PTPs). The

PTPs enter the interpeduncular fossa behind the mammillary bodies and supply the base of the oculomotor nerve, the posterior thalamus, the periventricular and median nuclei of the thalamus, the substantia nigra, the red nucleus, the midline midbrain structures, and the rostromedian floor of the fourth ventricle. Small branches are noted to extend anteriorly from the PTPs to supply the mammillary bodies and also the medial surface of the peduncles bilaterally.

In approximately 15% of individuals, one will note a hypoplastic P1 segment. This is frequently elongated, compared with its thicker counterpart. In addition, large perforators (0.5–1 mm) can arise from the hypoplastic segment, and fewer, smaller perforators may arise from the larger contralateral P1.

Perforators may come directly from the basilar artery itself just proximal to the bifurcation. At times, the PTPs may arise from a common vessel at the junction of the posterior communicating artery and the P1 segment. This vessel is distinct from the anterior thalamoperforators coming from the posterior communicating artery itself. One should note that the PTPs come from P1 and extend medially and superiorly in the interpuduncular fossa. However, the anterior thalamoperforators from the posterior communicating artery course laterally and superiorly. At times, the superior cerebellar artery can give rise proximally to a perforator that courses superiorly and anteromedially to enter the interpeduncular fossa.

## 8.3 Quadrigeminal Artery

The quadrigeminal artery (QA) most frequently arises from the P1 segment, usually 2 to 3 mm after the basilar bifurcation. It frequently gives off a small recurrent branch as a perforator into the interpeduncular fossa and may pierce the base of the third nerve, which it also supplies. The QA usually passes superior to the third nerve and medial to P1 but at times may pass inferior to the third nerve. As it extends around the peduncle, it parallels and is in close proximity to the posterior medial choroidal artery. On occasion, the QA may originate from the P2 segment immediately after the posterior communicating artery, but its absence is extremely rare. Its origin and distribution should be clearly distinguished from the posterior medial choroidal artery because the quadrigeminal artery may be double. The QA passes into the quadrigeminal cistern and terminates with branches extending over the surface of the superior colliculus and the upper portion of the inferior colliculus. It may give a small branch to the superior cerebellum.

## 8.4 Posterior Medial Choroidal Artery

The posterior medial choroidal artery (PMC) usually arises from the proximal P2 segment but on rare occasions may originate from the distal P1 segment. The PMC may be duplicated as it arises from P1 or P2. On occasion, there is an accessory posterior medial choroidal artery that arises from a P3 branch just distal to the main bifurcation of the P2 near or in the calcarine fissure. In the usual case, the PMC courses over the anterior and lateral peduncle hidden from view by the P2 segments of the posterior cerebral artery, extending into the ambient cisterns around to the quadrigeminal cistern and entering the third ventricle above the pineal gland. The PMC enters the roof of the third ventricle (tela choroidea) in the posterior portion of the cistern of the velum interpositum to supply the choroid plexus of the third ventricle, as well as branches piercing the choroidal fissure to supply the choroid plexus of the body and anterior horn of the lateral ventricle. The PMC, frequently, also supplies deep structures of the diencephalon. When an accessory posterior medial choroidal artery originates from the P3, it extends anteriorly from the anterior calcarine fissure to enter the third ventricle above the pineal gland into the velum interpositum.

## 8.5 Thalamogeniculate Perforators

The thalamogeniculate perforators (TGPs) are tiny vessels that arise from the distal segment of P2 and supply portions of the diencephalon. The TGPs are invariably present and may range from 2 to 12 in number. They frequently arise as individual vessels, and then branch into a multiplicity of smaller vessels that supply the deeper structures of the diencephalon. At times, the TGPs may arise from the segment of the P2 in the quadrigeminal cistern. These perforating arteries usually enter the brain between the medial and lateral geniculate bodies but could directly penetrate the medial geniculate, pulvinar, or lateral geniculate bodies.

## 8.6 Posterior Lateral Choroidal Arteries

The posterior lateral choroidal arteries (PLCs) have two distinct origins and distributions. There are usually two to four small PLCs originating directly from the P2 segment in the crural or ambient cisterns going directly to the choroid plexus in the temporal horn and trigone through the choroidal fissure and anastomosing with the anterior choroidal artery. The second and somewhat distinct component of the PLCs consists of one or two arteries that usually arise from the distal P2 or proximal P3 segments of the P2 and extend over the lateral and posterior edge of the pulvinar underneath the fornix, supplying branches to both structures. Usually, the more distal PLC is larger than the more proximal PLC. However, in general, if the anterior choroidal artery is very large, the PLC tends to be somewhat smaller.

## 8.7  Parietal Occipital Artery

The parietal occipital artery (PO) is invariably the main component of the bifurcation of the P2 in the calcarine sulcus. The PO imbeds in the calcarine sulcus, extending posteriorly, and then enters the parietal occipital sulcus to extend superiorly. The PO may give off the calcarine artery, as well as a posterior lateral choroidal artery and splenial artery. The PO frequently divides into two separate branches as it courses superiorly in the parietal-occipital sulcus.

## 8.8  Calcarine Artery

The calcarine artery (CA) is the other main branch of the bifurcation of the P2 deep in the calcarine sulcus. Its origin can be widely variable. At times, the CA can arise as a separate artery from the P2, extending up through the ambient cistern into the quadrigeminal cistern deep to the calcarine sulcus and back to the calcarine cortex. The CA that extends from the terminal bifurcation of the P2 toward the calcarine cortex may be tortuous and give off branches to the temporal occipital area, the cuneus, and the lingual gyrus. It should be noted that the CA can run deep in the calcarine sulcus or run superficially over the medial edge of the calcarine cortex.

## 8.9  Temporal Branches

The pattern of the temporal branches (TBs) from the P2 is variable. An anterior temporal branch from the P2 segment supplies the parahippocampal gyrus, and a smaller branch may extend anteriorly to supply the uncus. At times, the anterior temporal branch supplies a posterior lateral choroidal artery to the temporal horn. A more distal middle temporal branch also may give rise to a posterior lateral choroidal artery and/or an accessory posterior medial choroidal artery. The calcarine and parietal occipital branches can give rise to posterior temporal branches that extend out laterally and inferiorly.

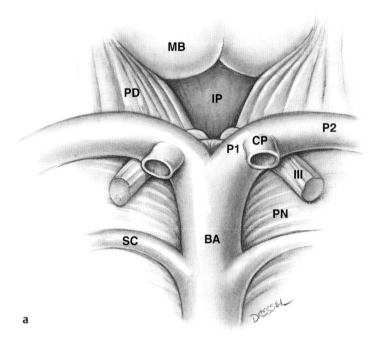

a

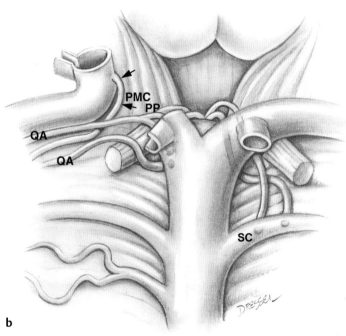

b

**Fig. 8.1** **(a)** Basilar artery bifurcation at the interpeduncular fossa (basic configuration).

BA   basilar artery
CP   posterior communicating artery
IP   interpeduncular fossa
MB   mammillary body
P1   posterior cerebral artery
P2   posterior cerebral artery
PD   peduncle
PN   pons
SC   superior cerebellar artery
III   third nerve

**Fig. 8.1** **(b)** There are two quadrigeminal arteries, one of which sends a retrograde perforator into the interpeduncular fossa. The left superior cerebellar artery (SC) sends perforators behind the P1 segment to the interpeduncular fossa.

PMC   posterior medial choroidal artery
PP     perforator
QA     quadrigeminal artery

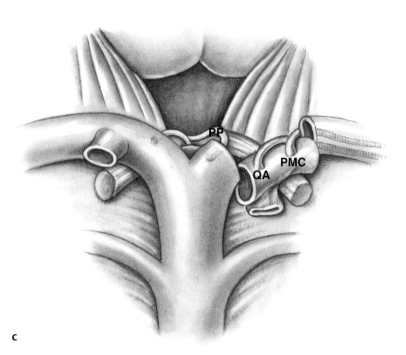

c

**Fig. 8.1  (c)** Note the relative position of the origin of the quadrigeminal artery and the posterior medial choroidal artery. The main perforators are from the proximal P1 segments.

PMC   posterior medial choroidal artery
PP      perforator
QA      quadrigeminal artery

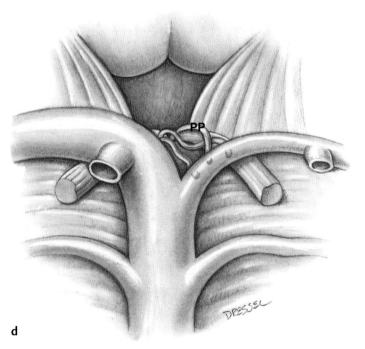

d

**Fig. 8.1  (d)** The P1 segment on the left is small in diameter, but the main perforators originate from this segment.

PP   perforator

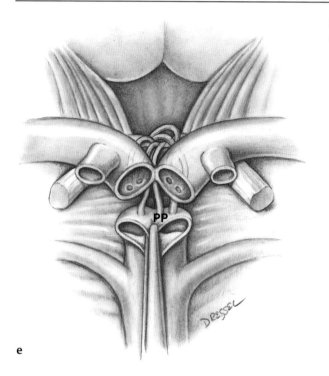

e

**Fig. 8.1** **(e)** The main perforators (PP) originate from the back wall of the basilar artery, just as it bifurcates into the two P1 segments.

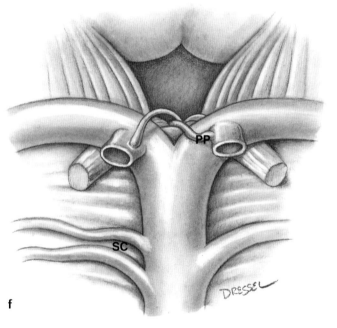

f

**Fig. 8.1** **(f)** In this less common variation, the perforators (PP) originate from the junction of the posterior communicating arteries with the P1 segments. Note the double superior cerebellar artery (SC) on the right side.

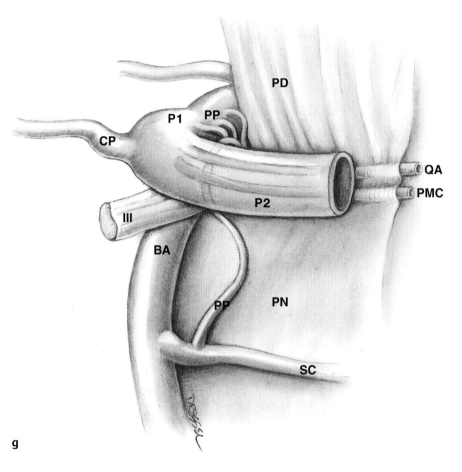

g

**Fig. 8.1   (g)** Left lateral view of the pons and peduncle. The posterior medial choroidal artery and the quadrigeminal artery are frequently sheathed in an arachnoid covering and can adhere closely to the peduncle. They are concealed in their course around the peduncle by the P2 segment.

| | |
|---|---|
| BA | basilar artery |
| CP | posterior communicating artery |
| P1 | posterior cerebral artery |
| P2 | posterior cerebral artery |
| PD | peduncle |
| PMC | posterior medial choroidal artery |
| PN | pons |
| PP | perforator |
| QA | quadrigeminal artery |
| SC | superior cerebellar artery |
| III | third nerve |

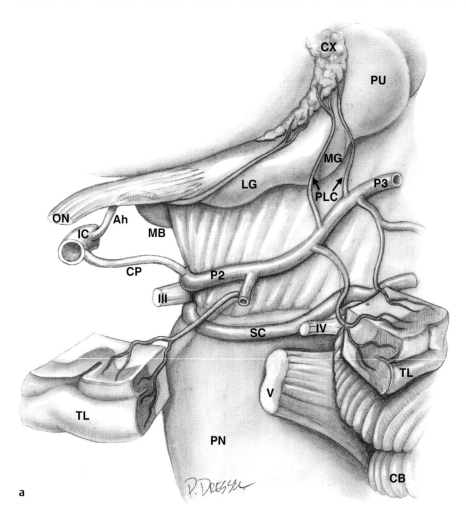

**Fig. 8.2** **(a)** View of the P2 segment as it encircles the peduncle to enter the quadrigeminal cistern posteriorly. Lateral view from the left side with removal of the left temporal lobe.

Ah   anterior choroidal artery
CB   cerebellum
CP   posterior communicating artery
CX   choroid plexus
IC   internal carotid artery
LG   lateral geniculate
MB   mammillary body
MG   medial geniculate
ON   optic nerve
P2   posterior cerebral artery
P3   posterior cerebral artery
PLC  posterior lateral choroidal artery
PN   pons
PU   pulvinar
SC   superior cerebellar artery
TL   temporal lobe
III  third nerve
IV   fourth nerve
V    fifth nerve

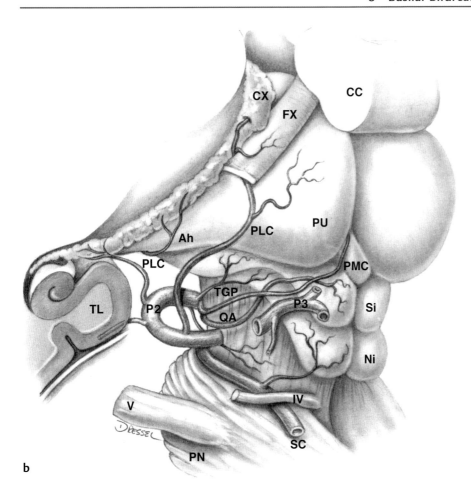

**Fig. 8.2   (b)** Left posterior lateral view with removal of the occipital parietal cerebrum.

Ah      anterior choroidal artery
CC      corpus callosum
CX      choroid plexus
FX      fornix
Ni      inferior colliculus
P2      posterior cerebral artery
P3      posterior cerebral artery
PLC     posterior lateral choroidal artery
PMC     posterior medial choroidal
        artery
PN      pons
PU      pulvinar
QA      quadrigeminal artery
SC      superior cerebellar artery
Si      superior colliculus
TGP     thalamo-geniculate perforators
TL      temporal lobe
IV      fourth nerve
V       fifth nerve

b

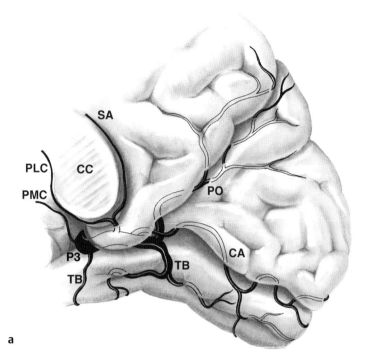

a

**Fig. 8.3** **(a)** Medial view of the right occipitoparietal region. Note that the posterior cerebral artery passes deep to the anterior calcarine fissure.

CA      calcarine artery
CC      corpus callosum
P3      posterior cerebral artery
PO      parieto-occipital artery
PLC     posterior lateral choroidal artery
SA      splenial artery
TB      temporal artery branch
PMC     accessory posterior medial choroidal artery

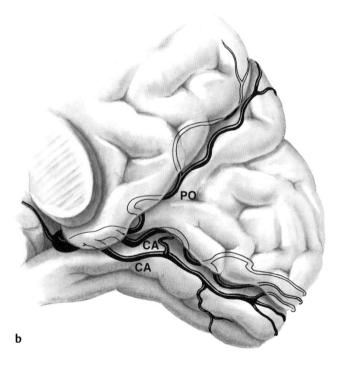

b

**Fig. 8.3** **(b–d)** Other variations of the calcarine artery. **(b)** There is a double origin of the calcarine artery: one branch coursing over the superior lip and the other over the inferior lip of the calcarine cortex, partially supplying other portions of the lingula.

CA   calcarine artery
PO   parieto-occipital artery

**Fig. 8.3   (c)** A single, large calcarine artery deep in the calcarine fissure giving off branches both superiorly and inferiorly.

CA   calcarine artery

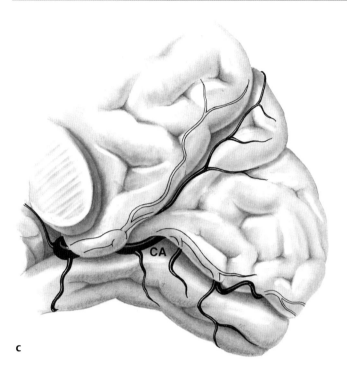

c

**Fig. 8.3   (d)** A complex bifurcation deep in the calcarine fissure with a looping of the calcarine artery and a separate posterior temporal branch that contributes to part of the inferior lip of the calcarine cortex.

CA   calcarine artery
TB   temporal artery branch

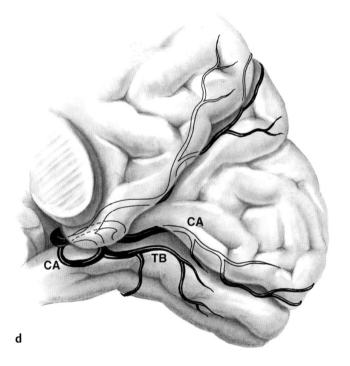

d

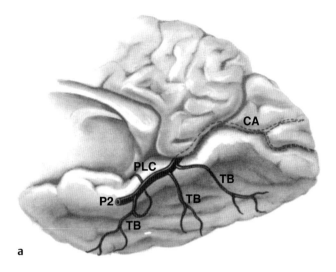

**Fig. 8.4** Variations of the P2 distributor to the temporal lobe. **(a)** Medial view of the right temporal lobe. This illustrates a retrograde posterior lateral choroidal artery from the anterior temporal branch.

CA   calcarine artery
P2   posterior cerebral artery
PLC   posterior lateral choroidal artery
TB   temporal artery branch

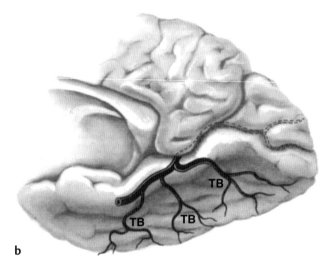

**Fig. 8.4** **(b)** This shows straightforward the anterior, middle, and posterior temporal branches.

TB   temporal artery branch

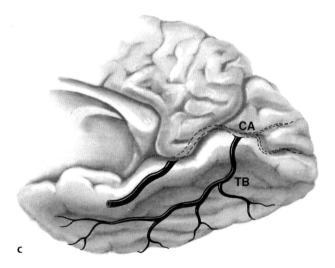

**Fig. 8.4** **(c)** Combined anterior, middle, and posterior cerebral branch coming off quite distal at the base of the calcarine artery, extending from posterior to anterior.

CA   calcarine artery
TB   temporal artery branch

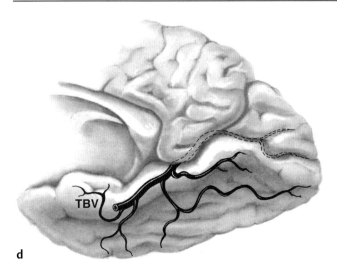

d

**Fig. 8.4** **(d)** There is a separate branch anteriorly to the uncus.

TBV    Temporal artery branch to uncus

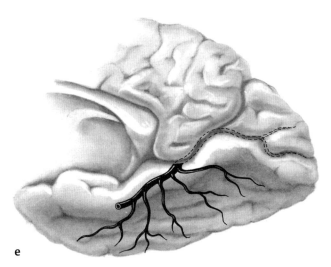

e

**Fig. 8.4** **(e)** There are five temporal branches.

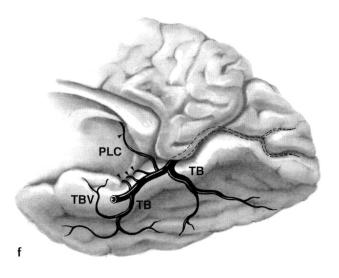

f

**Fig. 8.4** **(f)** There is a combined middle and anterior temporal branch with three proximal posterior lateral choroidal arteries (*arrowheads*) in addition to a larger, more distal posterior lateral choroidal artery.

PLC    posterior lateral choroidal artery
TB      temporal artery branch
TBV    temporal artery branch to uncus

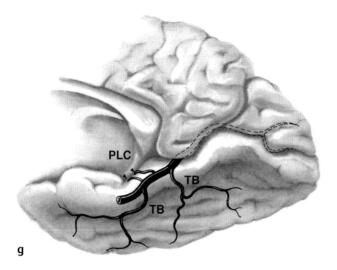

g

**Fig. 8.4** **(g)** A combined anterior middle temporal branch with only proximal posterior lateral choroidal arteries.

TB  temporal artery branch
PLC  posterior lateral choroidal artery

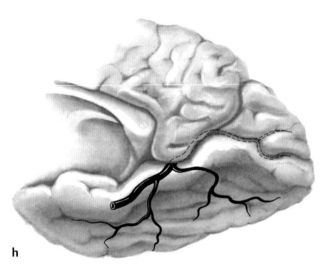

h

**Fig. 8.4** **(h)** Combined anterior and middle temporal branch with no proximal posterior lateral choroidal arteries.

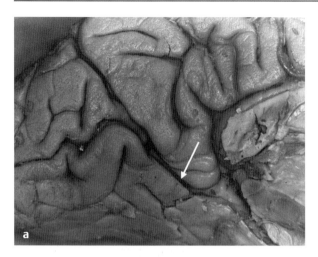

**Fig. 8.5** Variations and the linear configuration of the calcarine fissure. The variations and the configuration of the fissure indicate the general course of the artery within the fissure. **(a)** A double humped, ascending calcarine fissure (*arrow*) with the apex of the proximal hump going above the level of the corpus callosum.

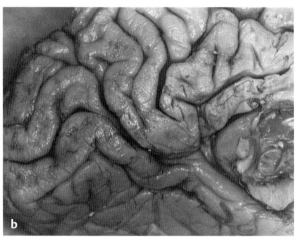

**Fig. 8.5** **(b)** A single hump in the calcarine fissure, again with the apex going above the level of the corpus callosum.

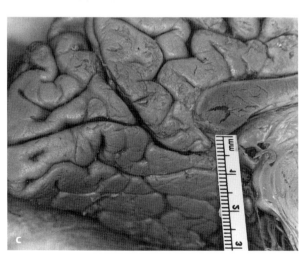

**Fig. 8.5** **(c)** A horizontal and flat calcarine fissure.

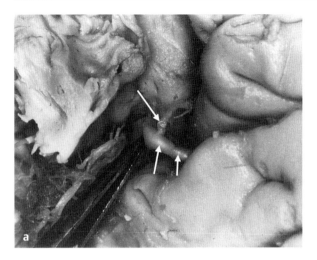

**Fig. 8.6** Medial view of the right hemisphere at the beginning of the calcarine fissure. Photos illustrate the origin of the splenial artery from the posterior cerebral artery. **(a)** The splenial artery (*single arrow*) originates a view millimeters prior to the entrance of the posterior cerebral artery (*double arrows*) into the calcarine fissure. The splenial artery then extends superiorly over the corpus callosum.

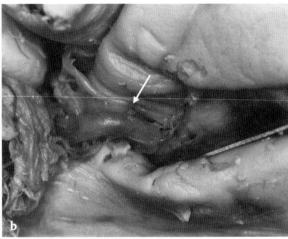

**Fig. 8.6** **(b)** The origin of the splenial artery (*arrow*) after the posterior cerebral artery enters deep into the initial portion of the calcarine fissure.

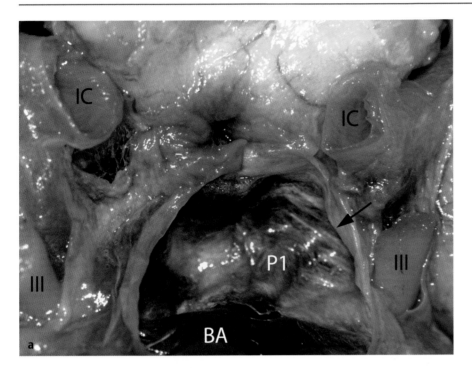

**Fig. 8.7** **(a)** Basal view of membrane of Liliequist opened (*arrow*) to expose the prepontine cistern. There is a secondary deep membrane covering the posterior cerebral artery (P1).

IC   internal carotid artery
BA   basilar artery
III   third nerve

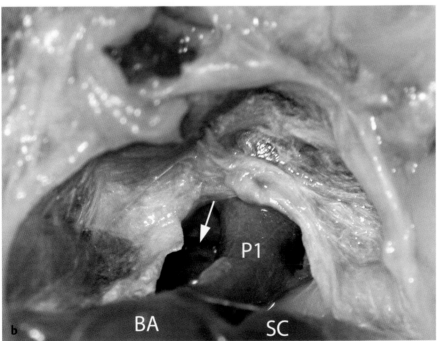

**Fig. 8.7** **(b)** Same specimen as **(a)**. The deep membrane is opened, revealing the P1 and deep to it the true interpeduncular fossa (*arrow*), which now communicates with the prepontine cistern.

BA   basilar artery
SC   superior cerebellar artery

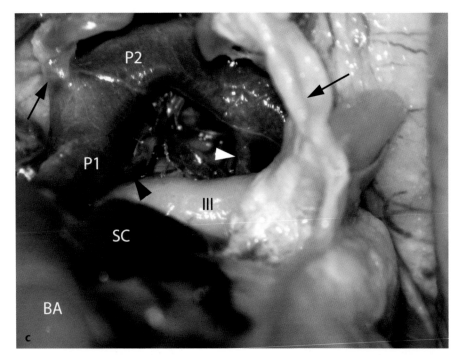

**Fig. 8.7** **(c)** Same specimen as **(a,b)**. Quadrigeminal artery arising from the posterior cerebral artery (P1) (*left arrowhead*); posterior medial choroidal artery arising from the posterior cerebral artery (P2) (*right arrowhead*).

BA  basilar artery
SC  superior cerebellar artery
III   third nerve
Upper left arrow  posterior communicating artery
Right arrow  edge of membrane of Liliequist

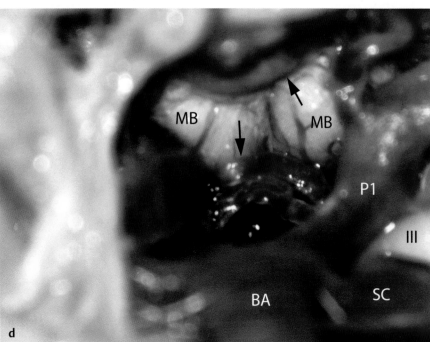

**Fig. 8.7** **(d)** Same specimen as **(a–c)**. The deep membrane is further stripped across the midline, exposing the interpeduncular fossa with perforators (*lower arrow*) and the mammillary bodies above. The edge of the tuber cinereum is visible (*upper arrow*).

P1  posterior cerebral artery
SC  superior cerebellar artery
MB  mammillary bodies
III   third nerve
BA  basilar artery

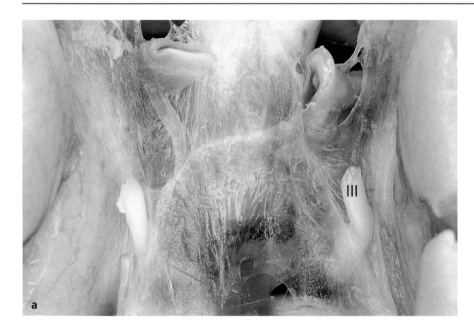

**Fig. 8.8   (a)** Another specimen with a view of the interpeduncular fossa with membrane of Liliequist (arachnoid membrane) intact.

III   third nerve

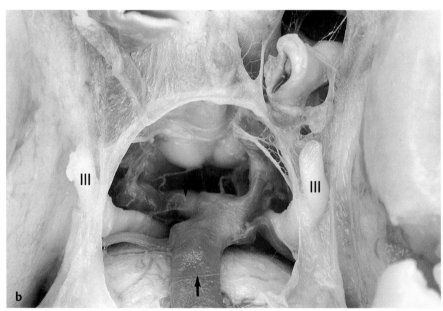

**Fig. 8.8   (b)** In contrast to **Fig. 8.7**, there is a large open cistern (Liliequist) after removing the membrane of Liliequist. Note that the third nerve exits the cistern in an arachnoid sheath just lateral to the edge of the membrane of Liliequist.

↑   basilar artery
▼   P1 segment
III   third nerve

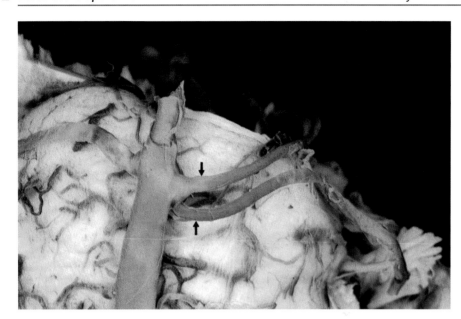

**Fig. 8.9** Double superior cerebellar artery (*arrows*).

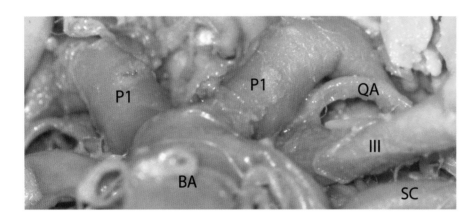

**Fig. 8.10** Ventral view of basilar bifurcation to illustrate origin of quadrigeminal artery (QA) from first portion of posterior cerebral artery (P1).

III   third nerve
BA   basilar artery
SC   superior cerebellar artery

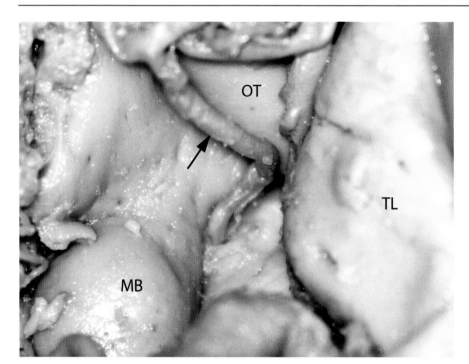

**Fig. 8.11**   Entry point of the premammillary artery (*arrow*).

MB   mammillary body
TL    temporal lobe (uncus)
OT   optic tract

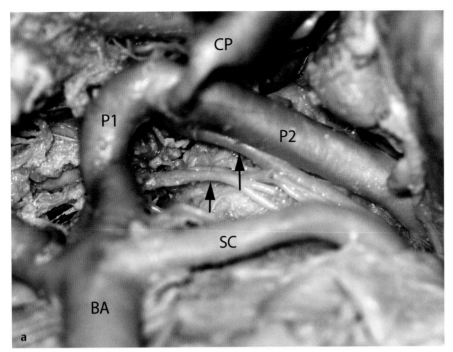

**Fig. 8.12** **(a)** Left posterior cerebral artery at the bifurcation of the basilar artery. The quadrigeminal artery (*left arrow*) from P1 and the posterior medial choroidal artery (*right arrow*) from P2.

BA   basilar artery
SC   superior cerebellar artery
CP   posterior communicating artery
P1, P2   posterior cerebral artery

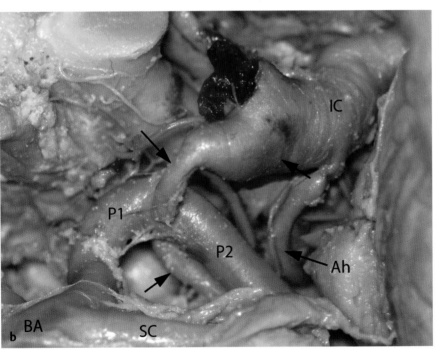

**Fig. 8.12** **(b)** Same specimen as **(a)**. P1 arising with a high anterior and superior "loop" from the basilar artery (BA). The posterior communicating artery (*left arrow*) arises from the internal carotid artery as an infundibulum (*upper right arrow*).

Ah   anterior choroidal artery
Left lower arrow   posterior medial choroidal artery
IC   internal carotid artery
SC   superior cerebellar artery
P1, P2   posterior cerebral artery

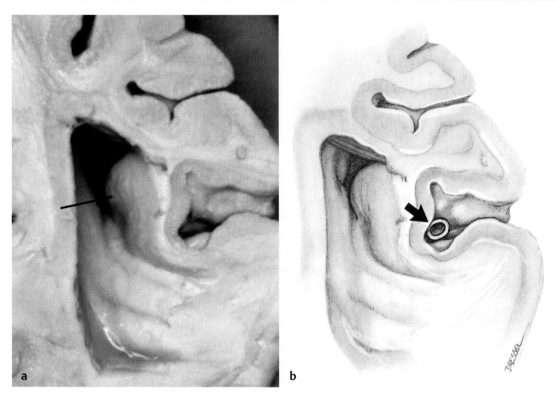

**Fig. 8.13** A coronal section through the right occipital hemisphere at the occipital horn, just behind the atrium of the lateral ventricle. **(a)** The calcar avis (*arrow*) is evident, bulging into the ventricular system. **(b)** This illustration shows the position of the calcarine artery (*arrow*) in relation to the calcar avis.

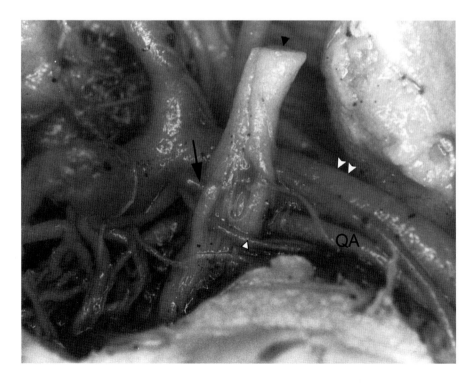

**Fig. 8.14** A close-up ventral view of the interpeduncular fossa on the left side of the brain stem, with the arachnoid stripped away, in the region of the left third nerve (*black arrowhead*). The quadrigeminal artery (QA) pierces (*arrow*) the third nerve on its course around the peduncle, paralleling and medial to the posterior cerebral artery (*white arrowheads*). In addition, there is a perforator (*white arrowhead*) at the base of the QA that is piercing the third nerve and coursing laterally.

## 8.10 Clinical Cases

### 8.10.1 Case 1

A middle-aged man presented with severe headaches for a few weeks. Workup, including computed tomography and lumbar puncture, was negative for subarachnoid hemorrhage. An angiogram confirmed the presence of a broad-based basilar apex aneurysm. Given the very broad neck and difficulty in preservation of both posterior cerebral artery (PCA) branches with a single stent, two stents in a **Y** configuration were placed sequentially into each PCA, and the aneurysm was subsequently coiled. The patient's headaches resolved, and the 3-month angiogram revealed no residual aneurysm.

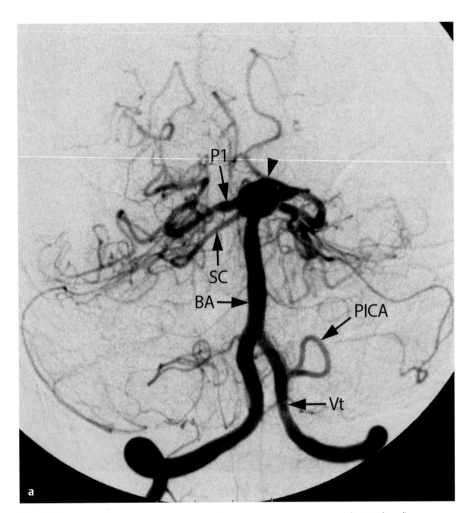

**Fig. 8.15**  **(a)** A 10-mm unruptured basilar artery apex aneurysm (*arrowhead*).

P1     posterior cerebral artery
SC     superior cerebellar artery
PICA   posterior inferior cerebellar artery
Vt     vertebral artery
BA     basilar artery

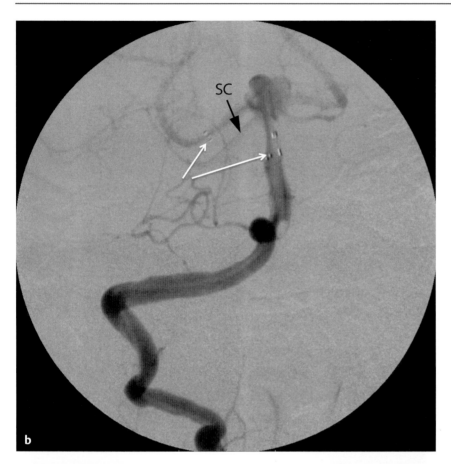

**Fig. 8.15** (*Continued*)  **(b)** A stent is placed in each posterior cerebral artery, making a **Y** configuration. The stent is visible in the basilar artery (*right arrow*). The end of the stent is seen in the right posterior cerebral artery (*left arrow*).

SC   superior cerebellar artery

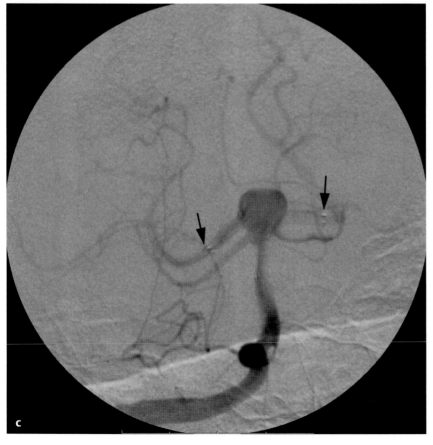

**Fig. 8.15** (*Continued*)  **(c)** A microcatheter is placed through an open cell in the stent into the left posterior cerebral artery (*right arrow*). Placement of a closed-cell stent is indicated (*left arrow*) in the right posterior cerebral artery.

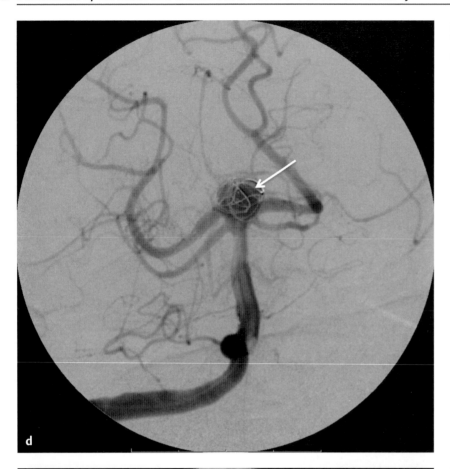

**Fig. 8.15** (*Continued*)   **(d)** Coils are placed in the aneurysm (*arrow*) through both stents.

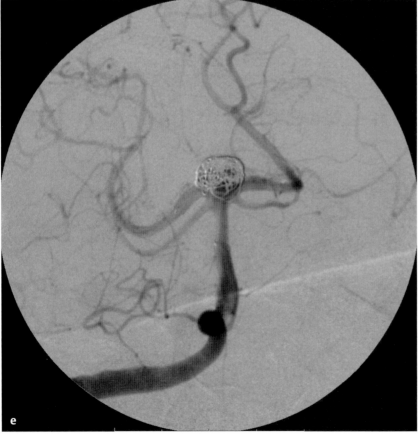

**Fig. 8.15** (*Continued*) **(e)** Coiling is completed.

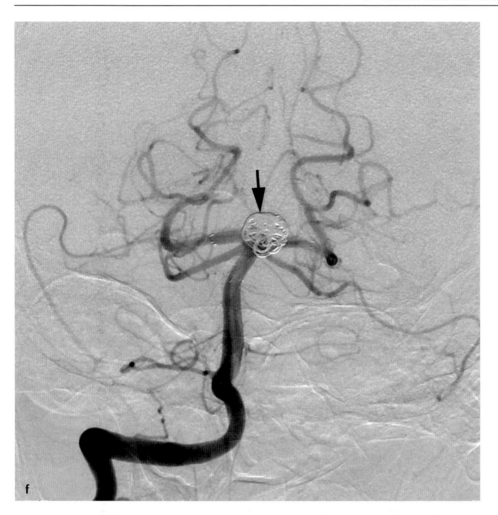

**Fig. 8.15** (*Continued*) **(f)** Three-month follow-up after coiling finds no residual aneurysm filling (*arrow*).

## 8.10.2 Case 2

A young man presented with right hemiparesis and visual dysfunction and headaches. Magnetic resonance imaging showed a partially thrombosed giant aneurysm compressing the left cerebral peduncle. Magnetic resonance angiography confirmed a giant left posterior cerebral artery (PCA) aneurysm. This fusiform aneurysm was treated by placing a single flow diverter across the aneurysm and jailing a microcatheter, which was used to coil the aneurysm. The patient's hemiparesis entirely resolved, and he was able to return to his occupation as a construction worker. Three-month follow-up angiography revealed complete patency of the PCA with obliteration of the aneurysm and resolution of peduncular mass effect.

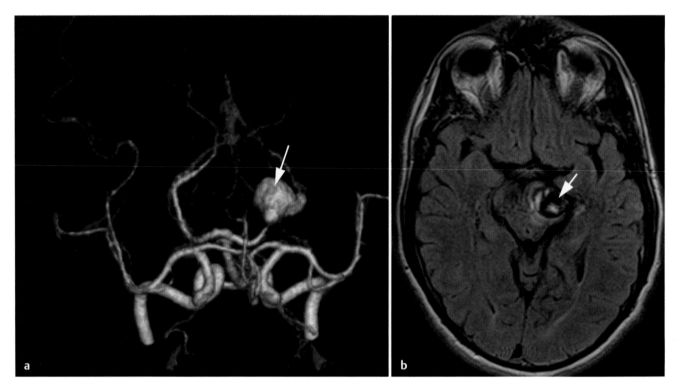

**Fig. 8.16** **(a)** Computed tomographic angiography shows a partially thrombosed left posterior cerebral artery aneurysm (*arrow*). **(b)** Unenhanced T1 magnetic resonance imaging of the brain shows a partially thrombosed aneurysm (*arrow*).

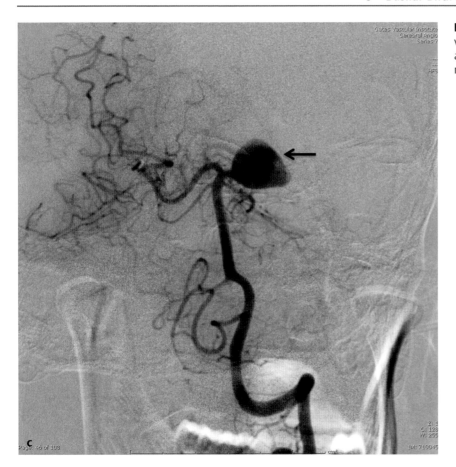

**Fig. 8.16** (*Continued*)   **(c)** Early-phase left vertebral angiography shows a dissecting aneurysm (*arrow*) of the left posterior cerebral artery.

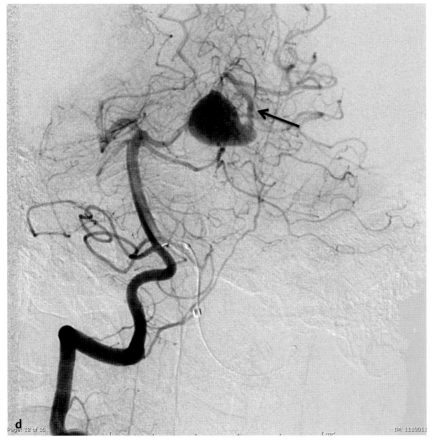

**Fig. 8.16**   **(d)** Late-phase left vertebral angiography shows delayed filling of the left posterior cerebral artery (*arrow*).

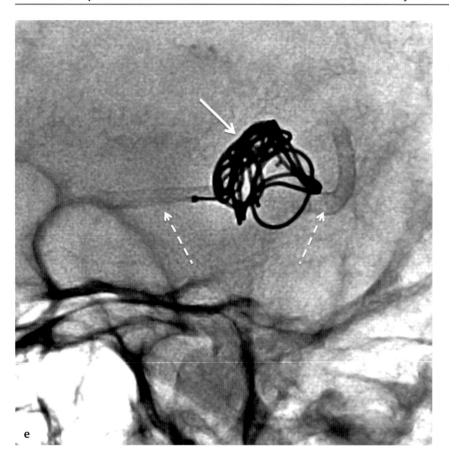

**Fig. 8.16** (*Continued*) **(e)** A stent diverter is inserted into the left posterior cerebral artery (*lower two arrows*), and there is partial coiling of the aneurysm (*upper arrow*).

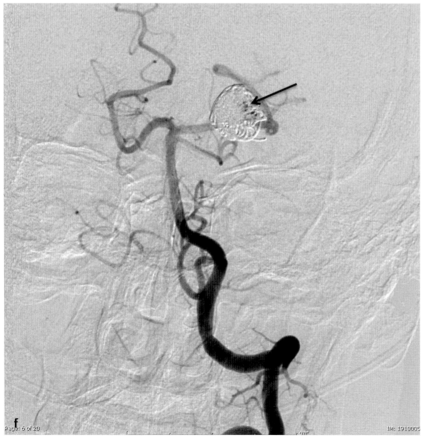

**Fig. 8.16** **(f)** End of coiling, with a small amount of filling of the aneurysm (*arrow*).

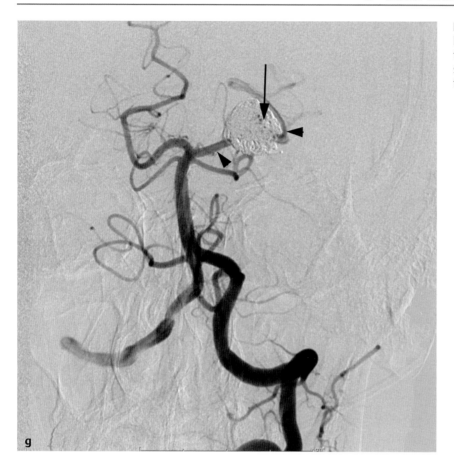

g

**Fig. 8.16** (*Continued*)   **(g)** At 3-month follow-up. Left vertebral angiography shows the left posterior cerebral artery is reconstructed (*arrowheads*). There is no residual filling of the aneurysm (*arrow*).

## 8.10.3 Case 3

A young woman presented with long-standing headaches and new-onset seizure. Workup revealed a left occipital arteriovenous malformation (AVM) supplied by branches from both the calcarine and parieto-occipital arteries. The patient underwent staged embolization of the AVM with liquid embolic agents with complete obliteration of the AVM.

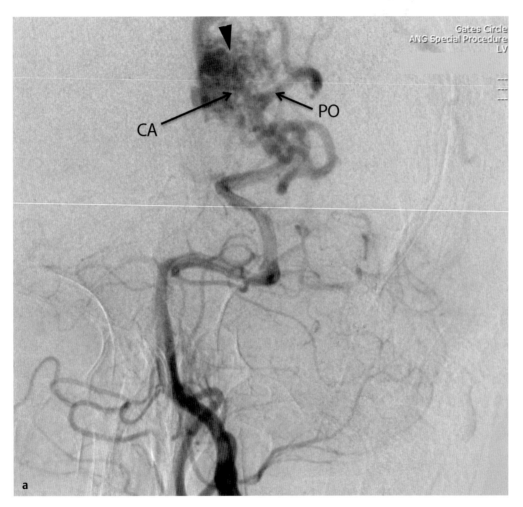

**Fig. 8.17** **(a)** Anteroposterior vertebral angiography shows a Spetzler–Martin grade 2 arteriovenous malformation (*arrowhead*) with contributions from the parieto-occipital artery (PO) and the calcarine artery (CA).

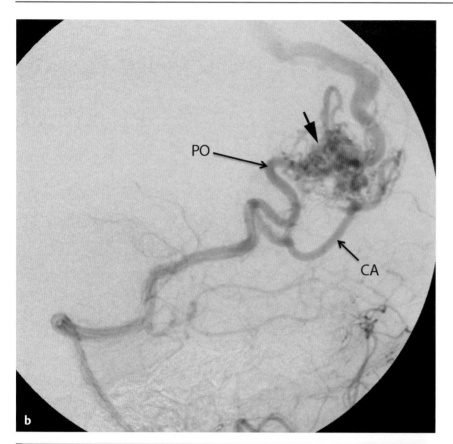

**Fig. 8.17** (*Continued*) **(b)** Lateral left vertebral angiography shows a Spetzler–Martin grade 2 arteriovenous malformation (*arrow*) with contributions from the parieto-occipital artery (PO) and the calcarine artery (CA).

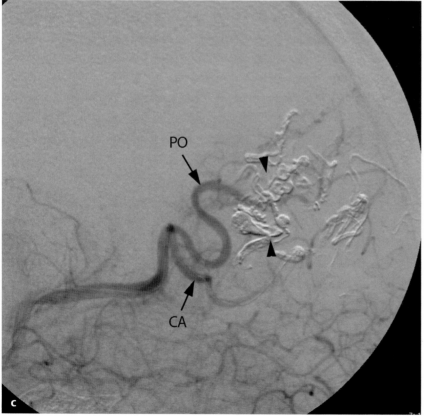

**Fig. 8.17** **(c)** Lateral left vertebral angiography shows embolization (*arrowheads*) via contributing vessels.

PO   parieto-occipital artery
CA   calcarine artery

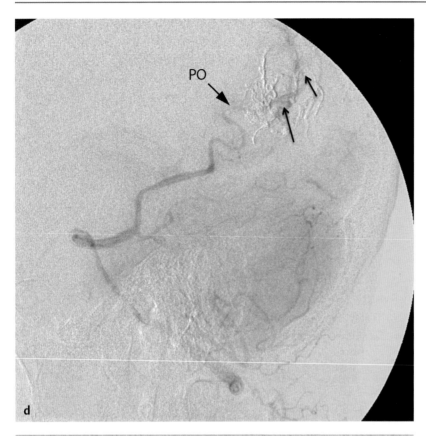

**Fig. 8.17** (*Continued*) **(d)** Left vertebral angiography at 1 year shows residual filling of the arteriovenous malformation from the parieto-occipital branch (PO), residual nidus (*left arrow*), and draining vein (*right arrow*).

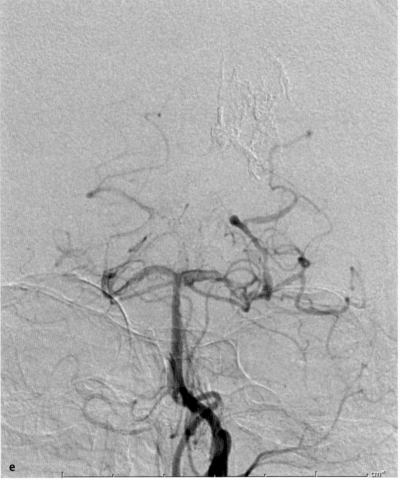

**Fig. 8.17** **(e)** Anteroposterior vertebral angiography at 4 years post–gamma knife radiation. The arteriovenous malformation does not fill.

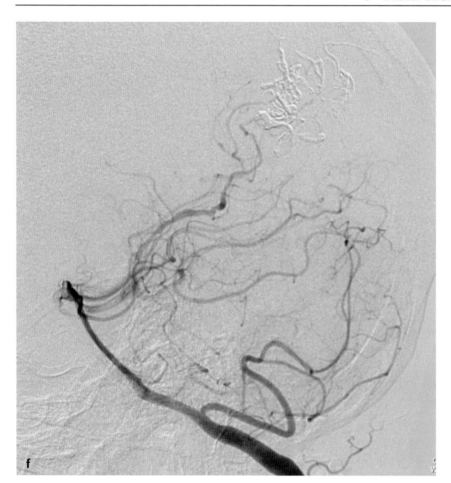

**Fig. 8.17** (*Continued*)  **(f)** Lateral left vertebral angiography at 4 years post–gamma knife radiation. The arteriovenous malformation does not fill.

## 8.10.4 Case 4

A middle-aged woman presented with a family history of aneurysms. She was noted on screening to harbor a basilar apex/superior cerebellar artery (SCA) aneurysm with a fetal right posterior cerebral artery (PCA). The SCA arose from the neck of the aneurysm. The patient was taken for clipping because endovascular preservation of the SCA branch was considered unlikely. The patient underwent a right orbitozygomatic craniotomy. The opticocarotid and carotico-oculomotor windows were developed after a wide Sylvian fissure exposure. A temporary clip was placed through the opticocarotid window, while the permanent clip was placed through the carotico-oculomotor window. The patient tolerated the procedure well without any deficits.

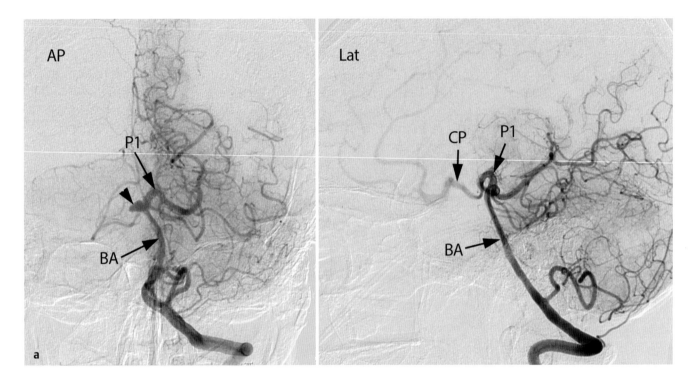

**Fig. 8.18** **(a)** Left vertebral angiography shows a basilar apex aneurysm (*arrowhead*).

P1   left posterior cerebral artery
CP   posterior communicating artery
BA   basilar artery

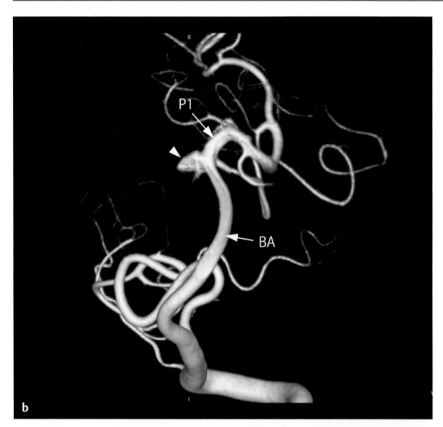

**Fig. 8.18** (*Continued*)   **(b)** Computed tomographic angiography reconstruction of **(a)** shows the aneurysm (*arrowhead*).

P1   left posterior cerebral artery
BA   basilar artery

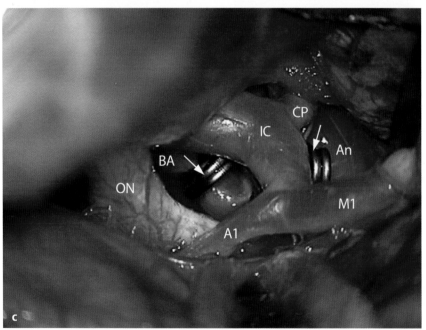

**Fig. 8.18**   **(c)** Operative view of right orbitozygomatic approach to the basilar apex aneurysm. A temporary clip is seen on the BA (*left arrow*), as well as a clip on the neck of the aneurysm (*right arrow*).

ON   right optic nerve
IC    right internal carotid artery
CP   right posterior communicating artery
BA   basilar artery
A1   right anterior cerebral artery
M1   right middle cerebral artery
An   aneurysm dome

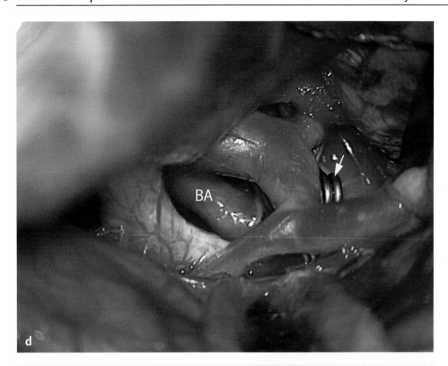

**Fig. 8.18** (*Continued*) **(d)** Temporary clip has been removed from the basilar artery (BA), and the permanent aneurysm clip is in place (*arrow*).

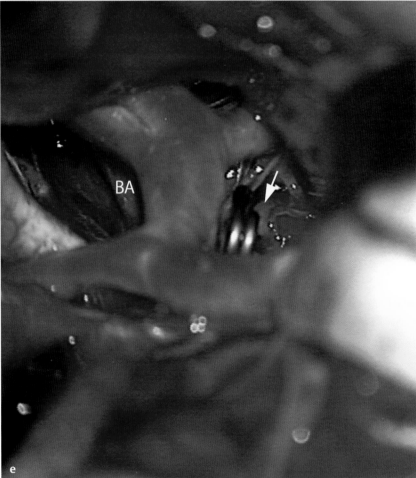

**Fig. 8.18** **(e)** A more lateral view of **(d)** with the permanent aneurysm clip in place. The base of the aneurysm just distal to the clip is in view (*arrow*).

BA   basilar artery

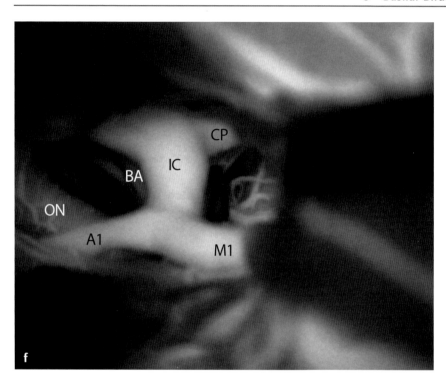

**Fig. 8.18** (*Continued*) **(f)** Intraoperative indocyanine angiography shows no filling of the aneurysm.

ON  optic nerve
BA  basilar artery
IC  internal carotid artery
CP  posterior communicating artery
A1  anterior cerebral artery
M1  middle cerebral artery

## Clinical Pearls

- During surgical exposure of the basilar bifurcation from a transsylvian approach, the posterior communicating artery (PCom) serves as an important landmark. It can be followed posteriorly through the thickened arachnoid membrane of Liliequist, which, when opened, exposes the P1 and P2 junction. The P1 can then be followed medially to expose the basilar terminus. The PCom typically travels medial and superior to the oculomotor nerve.

- Although endovascularly these perforators are easy to avoid, it is precisely their protection and preservation that complicates surgical approaches. Two major windows are used during surgical management of basilar apex aneurysms, namely the carotico-optic and the corotico-oculomotor windows. As the names suggest, they lie between the named structures. Frequently, both need to be exposed to adequately exert proximal control on the basilar artery, as well as identify the contralateral posterior cerebral artery, superior cerebellar artery, and third nerve.

- During the penultimate hippocampal resection during a medial hippocampectomy, the posterior cerebral artery (PCA) is exposed to injury. This risk can be reduced through a subpial dissection plane. A subtemporal approach can also be used for aneurysms of the basilar apex and P1/P2 junction. This approach frequently requires greater cerebrospinal fluid drainage and retraction of the temporal lobe over the incisura.

- Aneurysms of the P2/P3 junction can be hard to expose through a straightforward, subtemporal approach, because the vessel starts climbing more superiorly as it approaches the calcarine sulci. In these cases, endovascular treatment offers a much more straightforward approach. However, if surgical exposure is needed, it may be easier through a supracerebellar transtenorial approach.

### Posterior Thalamoperforators

- These perforators are the most important limiting factors during surgical exposure to the basilar apex. The anatomy is deep and is hidden behind vital structures, such as the optic nerve and tract, internal carotid artery, and posterior communicating artery vessels, and frequently, the posterior clinoid process. In addition, injury to some of these perforators, such as the named artery of Percheron, may result in major deficits, which can be bilateral, as well as affecting consciousness because of ischemia to the midline raphe and reticular activating system in the rostral midbrain.

  In sharp contrast, endovascular intervention is ideal because of a relatively straight basilar artery leading to bifurcation, significantly better visualization, and an ability to protect these key branches through adjunctive endovascular techniques, such as stents and balloons.

  The posterior medial choroidal artery originates from the parieto-occipital branch of the posterior cerebral artery (P3), it extends anteriorly from the anterior calcarine fissure to enter the third ventricle above the pineal gland into the velum interpositum.

- Catheterization and embolization of this branch during treatment of arteriovenous malformations carries a similar risk as other perforators because of terminal branches that supply, beyond the choroid plexus, the deep nuclei of the midbrian and thalamus. These branches are the most commonly involved, supplying the fistulas that feed vein of Galen malformations.

- The calcarine branch supplies the primary visual cortex along the banks of the calcarine sulcus and frequently anastomoses with the terminal branches of the middle cerebral artery. These anastomoses can be rich enough that a balloon test occlusion can be performed in an awake patient to test if a proximal occlusion will result in hemianopsia.

### Temporal Branches

- Temporal branches from the posterior cerebral artery are critical collaterals to the middle cerebral artery distribution, which allow for the penumbra to survive following M1 occlusions.

# 9  Vertebral and Basilar Arteries

The vertebral artery at the cranial base enters the foramen magnum, and the vertebral arteries join one another to form the lower basilar artery at the pontomedullary junction. Initially, the extracranial portion of the vertebral artery lies within the foramen of the transverse processes of the axis and atlas. It passes through the foramen of the second cervical (axis) transverse process and proceeds superiorly through the foramen of the transverse process of the atlas (first cervical vertebra). The vertebral artery then passes medially over the superior arch of the atlas in a groove posterior to the superior articular surface of the atlas. As the vertebral artery ascends from the axis to the atlas, it becomes encased in a venous plexus and venous cavity. From this venous plexus, the condylar emissary vein goes through the condylar foramen to communicate with the jugular bulb. The vertebral artery at the cranial base, in its extradural course, has muscular branches, radicular branches, and dural branches. The muscular branches of the vertebral artery can collateralize extensively with the muscular branches of the occipital artery, and, in this fashion, the external carotid circulation and vertebral artery circulation may form "dangerous anastomoses." The branches to the dura from the vertebral artery may originate extradurally and then penetrate the dura with the vertebral artery, or originate from the vertebral artery just after it enters the intradural compartment. The dural branches and the posterior spinal branch may have a common stem. The vertebral artery in its extradural course between the axis and atlas may give off a radicular branch that follows the C2 nerve root to penetrate the dura and supply the posterior aspect of the spinal cord.

## 9.1 Posterior Inferior Cerebellar Artery

The posterior inferior cerebellar artery has a variable origin from the intradural vertebral artery. It may originate from the vertebral artery just after its penetration of the dura or in close proximity to the vertebrobasilar junction. It may be absent and, if so, is usually replaced by an enlarged anterior inferior cerebellar artery that supplies the territory of the inferior and medial cerebellum, as well as the usual distribution of the anterior inferior cerebellar artery. The posterior inferior cerebellar artery has an anterior medullary segment, a lateral medullary segment, and a posterior medullary segment. As the posterior inferior cerebellar artery loops behind the medulla into its posterior medullary segment, its relationship to the tonsils of the cerebellum and its curvature posteriorly and inferiorly along the medial cerebellum are quite variable. It usually gives a branch to the choroid plexus in the inferior and posterior fourth ventricle. In conjunction with the vertebral artery, the posterior inferior cerebellar artery supplies critical perforators to the regions posterior and inferior to the olivary nucleus. The posterior inferior cerebellar artery, as it courses over the tonsils in its final distribution, gives branches to the vermis and the medial and inferior cerebellar hemispheres, and it collateralizes with the anterior inferior cerebellar artery and the superior cerebellar artery over the surface of the cerebellar hemispheres. The branching of the posterior inferior cerebellar artery is quite variable and depends somewhat on its course in relation to the cerebellar tonsils.

## 9.2 Anterior Spinal Artery

The anterior spinal artery originates from the vertebral artery just prior to its junction to form the basilar artery. The configuration of the anterior spinal artery is quite variable. The anterior spinal artery may be absent on one side or may form a bridging network with its partner from the opposite vertebral artery. Even though the vertebral artery may be very hypoplastic, the ipsilateral anterior spinal artery may be quite large and, in fact, may be the only significant anterior spinal artery supply to the spinal cord.

## 9.3 Vertebrobasilar Junction

The vertebrobasilar junction is formed by the joining of the two vertebral arteries into the lower basilar artery. At this point, at the area designated as the foramen cecum, as the medulla joins the pons, this critical anatomical pocket receives perforators from the superior surface of the lower basilar artery to penetrate the pontomedullary junction.

## 9.4 Anterior Inferior Cerebellar Artery

The anterior inferior cerebellar artery originates from the lower portion of the basilar artery or at the lateral portion of the vertebrobasilar junction. The artery runs within the cerebellopontine angle and is in close proximity to the facial and auditory nerves. The internal auditory artery arises from the anterior inferior cerebellar artery. If the anterior inferior cerebellar artery is a combined artery including the distribution of the posterior inferior cerebellar artery, its configuration will obviously be drastically altered. The distribution of the posterior inferior cerebellar artery territory from a common trunk with the anterior inferior cerebellar artery may come as an early branch from the anterior inferior cerebellar artery or as a more distal branch in the lateral medullary segment. The anterior inferior cerebellar artery distributes its branches not only in the cerebellopontine angle but also to the inferior and posterior cerebellar hemisphere below the horizontal fissure. The anterior inferior cerebellar artery anastomoses superiorly with the superior cerebellar artery. The anterior inferior cerebellar artery also distributes perforators to the area superior and posterior to the olivary nucleus.

## 9.5 Superior Cerebellar Artery

The superior cerebellar artery originates from the upper basilar artery just inferior to the origin of the third nerve. The superior cerebellar artery may be duplicated on either or both sides. When duplicated, the inferior superior cerebellar artery supplies the lateral and superior cerebellum, whereas the more superior duplicate supplies the more medial cerebellum and the vermis. When the superior cerebellar artery is single, its initial bifurcation is variable and may take place in the ambient or quadrigeminal cistern. In either case, the more medial branch supplies the superior and medial cerebellum and the superior vermis. In the quadrigeminal cistern, the superior cerebellar artery can become quite tortuous, and the fourth nerve can be seen beneath and anterior to the convoluted branches of the superior cerebellar artery. In general, the superior cerebellar artery supplies the area of the cerebellum superior to the horizontal fissure and then collateralizes with the anterior inferior cerebellar artery and the posterior inferior cerebellar artery. The superior cerebellar artery in the quadrigeminal cistern also supplies the inferior colliculus.

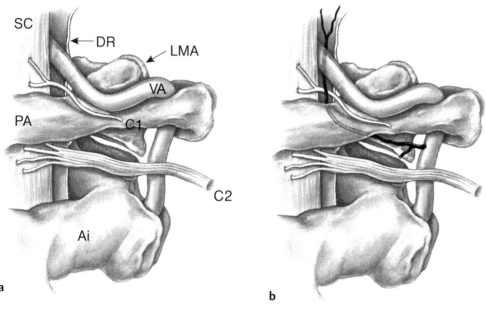

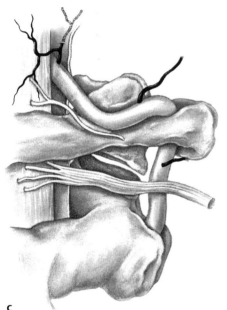

**Fig. 9.1** **(a)** A posterior view of the atlas and axis as the vertebral artery courses superiorly and medially to penetrate the dura and courses anteriorly to the cervicomedullary junction. **(b–c)** The variations of the branch of the vertebral artery that penetrates and supplies the posterior fossa dura. Frequently, the same vessel that penetrates the dura gives off a small twig that supplies the posterior spinal cord.

Ai     axis
C1     first cervical root
C2     second cervical root
DR     dura
LMA   lateral mass of atlas
PA     posterior arch of atlas
VA     vertebral artery
SC     spinal cord

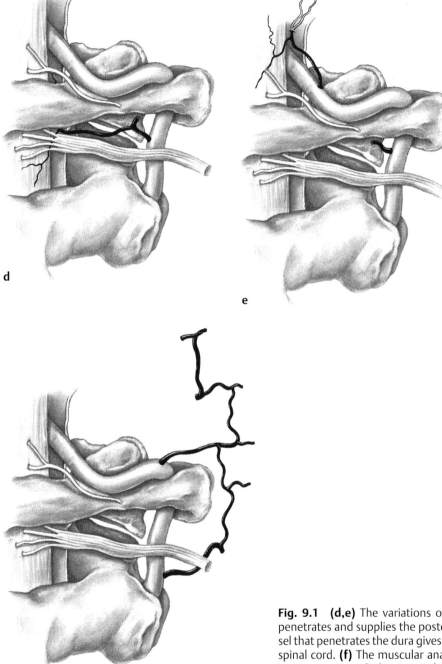

d

e

f

**Fig. 9.1** **(d,e)** The variations of the branch of the vertebral artery that penetrates and supplies the posterior fossa dura. Frequently, the same vessel that penetrates the dura gives off a small twig that supplies the posterior spinal cord. **(f)** The muscular anastomoses in the neck that superiorly can communicate with the occipital artery.

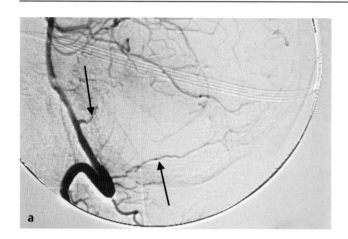

**Fig. 9.2**  **(a)** A lateral vertebral arteriogram with an occlusion of the posterior inferior cerebellar artery (*upper arrow*) just at the beginning of the posterior medullary portion. This allows one to see clearly the meningeal branch (*lower arrow*) arising from the vertebral artery.

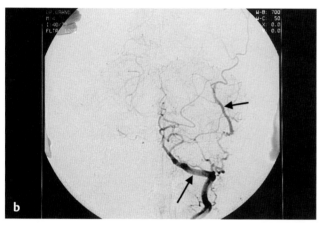

**Fig. 9.2**  **(b)** A left vertebral (*lower arrow*) angiogram showing collateralization to the occipital artery (*upper arrow*), illustrating a "dangerous anastomosis."

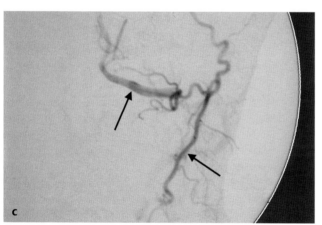

**Fig. 9.2**  **(c)** An arteriogram of the external carotid circulation with selective catherization of the left occipital artery (*right arrow*) and collateralization into the left vertebral artery (*left arrow*), again illustrating a "dangerous anastomosis."

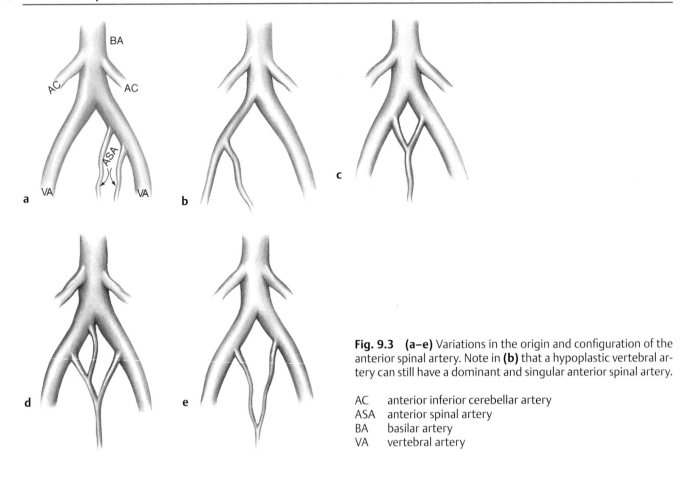

**Fig. 9.3 (a–e)** Variations in the origin and configuration of the anterior spinal artery. Note in **(b)** that a hypoplastic vertebral artery can still have a dominant and singular anterior spinal artery.

AC     anterior inferior cerebellar artery
ASA    anterior spinal artery
BA     basilar artery
VA     vertebral artery

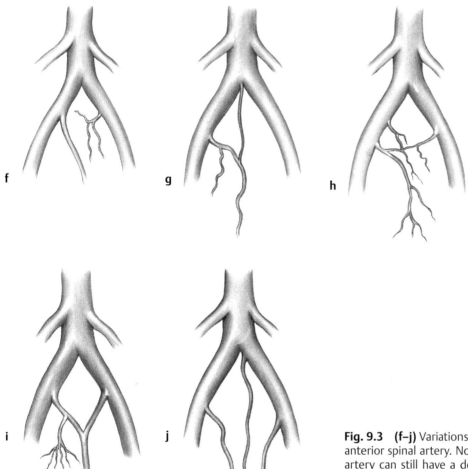

**Fig. 9.3** **(f–j)** Variations in the origin and configuration of the anterior spinal artery. Note in **(b)** that a hypoplastic vertebral artery can still have a dominant and singular anterior spinal artery.

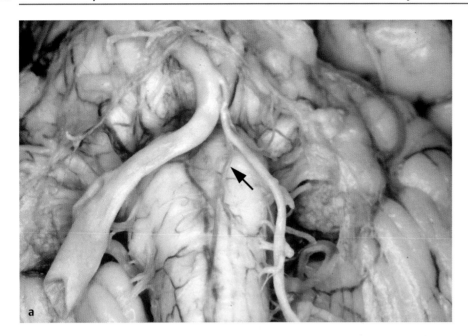

**Fig. 9.4 (a)** Marked disparity between the sizes of the two vertebral arteries, but the single anterior spinal artery (*arrow*) arises from the hypoplastic vertebral artery.

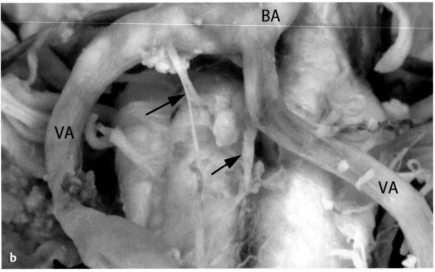

**Fig. 9.4 (b)** Anterior spinal arteries (*arrows*) originating from each vertebral artery (VA). Note that the larger anterior spinal artery (*right arrow*) arises from the smaller vertebral artery.

BA   basilar artery

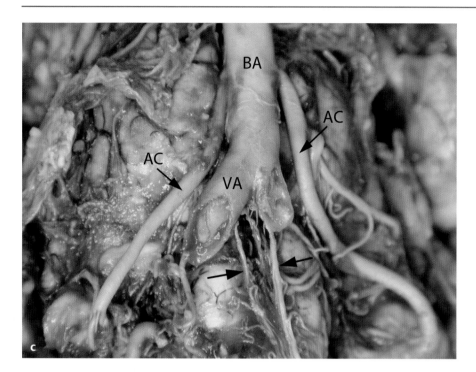

**Fig. 9.4 (c)** Anterior spinal arteries (*arrows*) arise from each vertebral artery.

BA   basilar artery
VA   vertebral artery
AC   anterior inferior cerebellar artery

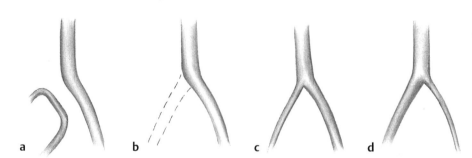

**Fig. 9.5 (a–d)** Variations in the configuration of the two vertebral arteries as they join the basilar artery.

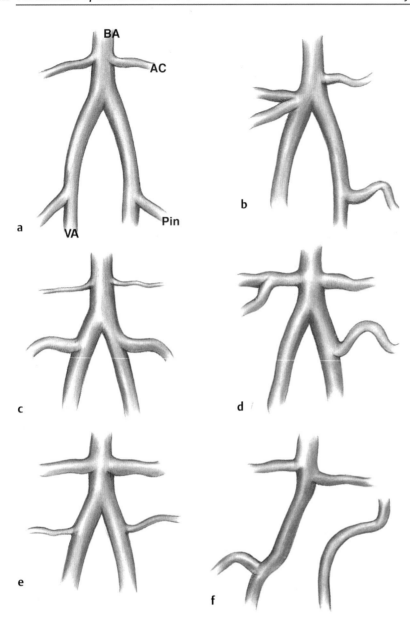

**Fig. 9.6 (a–f)** Variations in the configuration and relationship of the anterior inferior cerebellar artery and the posterior inferior cerebellar artery.

AC   anterior inferior cerebellar artery
BA   basilar artery
Pin  posterior inferior cerebellar artery
VA   vertebral artery

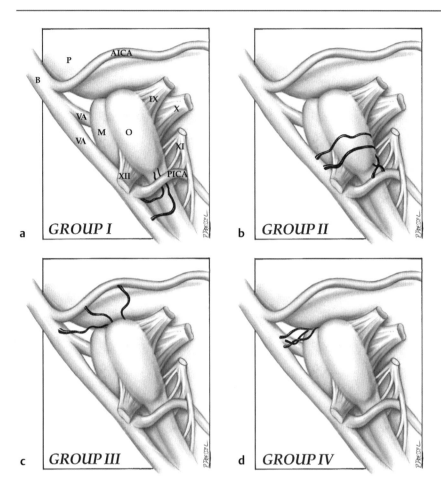

a **GROUP I**

b **GROUP II**

c **GROUP III**

d **GROUP IV**

**Fig. 9.7** **(a)** Perforators from the proximal vertebral artery penetrate the lateral medullary area in the posterior olivary sulcus. **(b)** Perforators arise from the posterior inferior cerebellar artery and more distal vertebral artery to penetrate the posterior olivary sulcus. **(c)** Perforators from the vertebrobasilar junction and the anterior inferior cerebellar artery penetrate the superior olivary groove. **(d)** Perforators from the vertebrobasilar junction penetrate the region of the foramen cecum.

AICA    anterior inferior cerebellar artery
B    basilar artery
M    medulla
O    olive
P    pons
PICA    posterior inferior cerebellar artery
VA    vertebral artery
IX    ninth nerve
X    tenth nerve
XI    eleventh nerve
XII    twelfth nerve

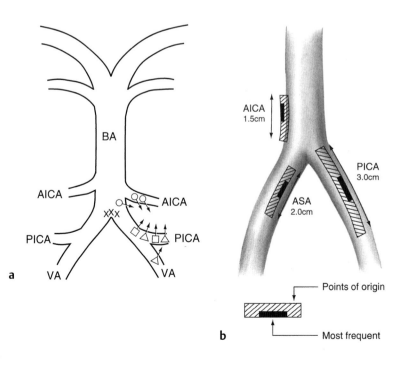

a

b

**Fig. 9.8** **(a)** illustrates the four groups of lower brainstem perforating arteries: Triangle 9–7A (Group 1); Square 9–7B (Group 2); Circle 9–7C (Group 3); X 9–7D (Group 4). **(b)** The relative frequency of the origin of the anterior spinal artery from the vertebral artery and the origin of the posterior inferior cerebellar artery from the vertebral artery. The relative frequency and points of origin of the anterior inferior cerebellar artery are also shown.

AICA    anterior inferior cerebellar artery
ASA    anterior spinal artery
BA    basilar artery
PICA    posterior inferior cerebellar artery
VA    vertebral artery

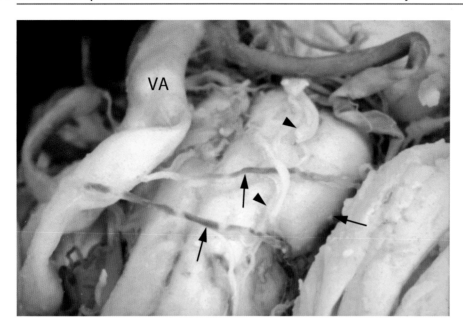

**Fig. 9.9** Perforators (*left arrows*) arising from the vertebral artery (VA). See **Fig. 9.7b**.

Right arrow    olive
Arrowheads    rootlets of the
                hypoglossal nerve

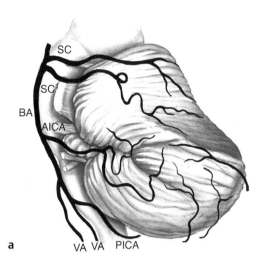

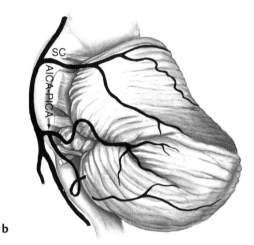

**Fig. 9.10 (a–c)** Lateral view of the left side of the cerebellum and brainstem. Variations in the configuration of the superior cerebellar artery, anterior inferior cerebellar artery, and posterior inferior cerebellar artery are shown.

AICA   anterior inferior cerebellar artery
BA      basilar artery
PICA   posterior inferior cerebellar artery
SC      superior cerebellar artery
SC$^1$    superior cerebellar artery (inferior duplicate)
VA      vertebral artery

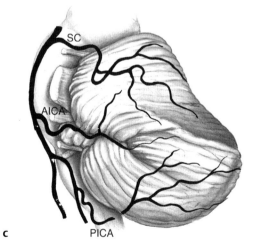

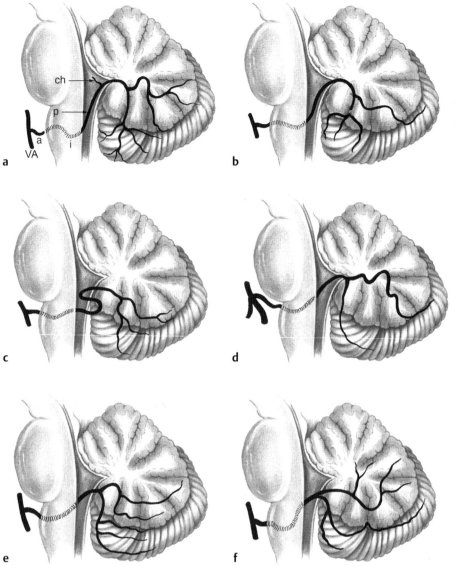

**Fig. 9.11** **(a–f)** Medial view of the right cerebellar hemisphere transsected through the vermis. **(a,g)** The origin of the choroidal artery.

a    PICA, anterior medullary segment
i    PICA, lateral medullary segment
ch   choroidal artery
p    PICA, posterior medullary segment
VA   vertebral artery

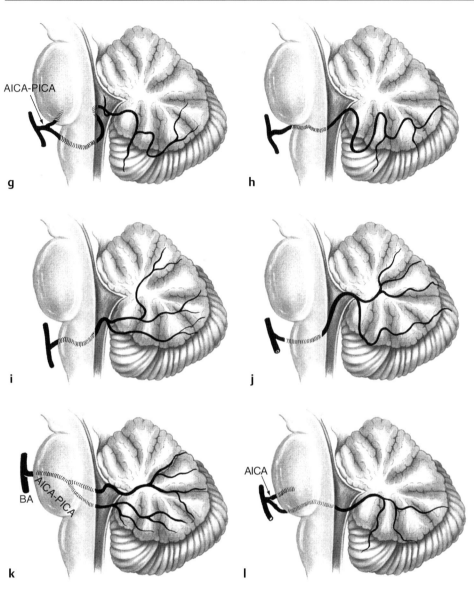

**Fig. 9.11** **(g–l)** Medial view of the right cerebellar hemisphere transsected through the vermis. **(g,k,l)** Variations in configuration of the posterior inferior cerebellar artery as it arises from the vertebral artery and the common origin of the anterior inferior cerebellar artery and posterior inferior cerebellar artery. **(a,g)** The origin of the choroidal artery.

ch   choroidal artery
PICA   posterior medullary segment
VA   vertebral artery
AICA   anterior inferior cerebellar artery
BA   basilar artery

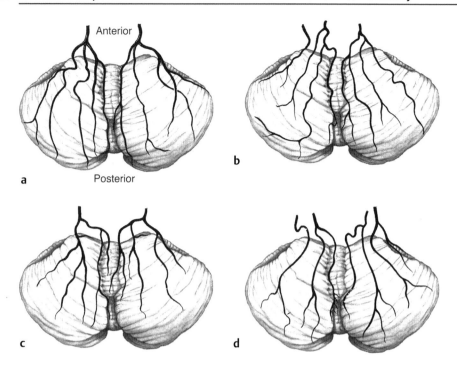

**Fig. 9.12** Superior view of the cerebellum. **(a)** Trifurcation of the superior cerebellar artery and division of blood supply into the medial, central, and lateral cerebellum. **(b)** On the left of the figure, the superior cerebellar artery is duplicated with the inferior duplicate supplying the lateral cerebellum. **(c)** An early bifurcation of the superior cerebellar artery. On the left of the figure, the more lateral branch provides the dominant blood supply to the cerebellar hemisphere, whereas on the right of the figure, the medial branch provides the dominant blood supply to the cerebellar hemisphere. **(d)** Bilateral double superior cerebellar arteries with the superior duplicate supplying the more medial cerebellar hemisphere, and the inferior originating superior cerebellar artery supplying the more lateral cerebellar hemisphere.

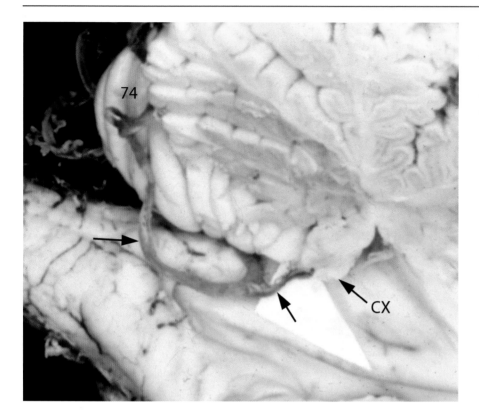

**Fig. 9.13** Sagittal cut-away of cerebellar hemisphere. The posterior inferior cerebellar artery (*left arrow*) supplies a branch (*right arrow*) to the choroid plexus (CX) of the fourth ventricle and then proceeds caudally and superiorly over the tonsil (74).

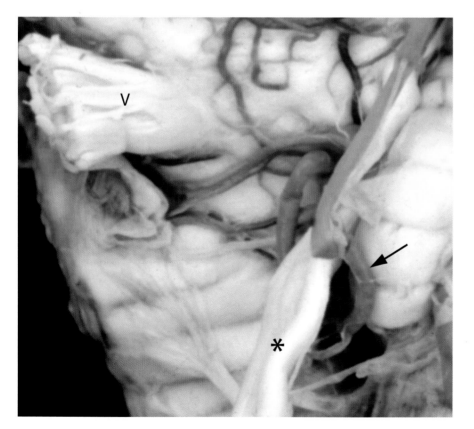

**Fig. 9.14** Lateral view of the left pontomedullary junction with a branch of the anterior inferior cerebellar artery (*arrow*) looped around the seventh to eighth nerve complex (*).

V    fifth nerve

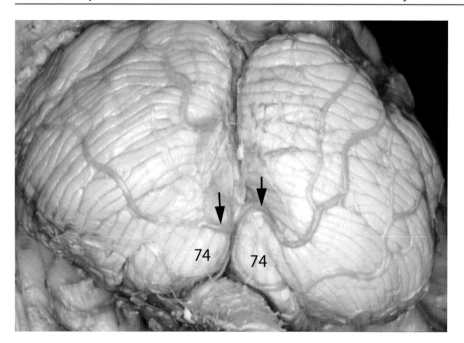

**Fig. 9.15** Posterior view of the cerebellar hemispheres showing the posterior inferior cerebellar artery on each side (*arrows*) emerging in the midline on the undersurface of the cerebellum.

74   tonsils

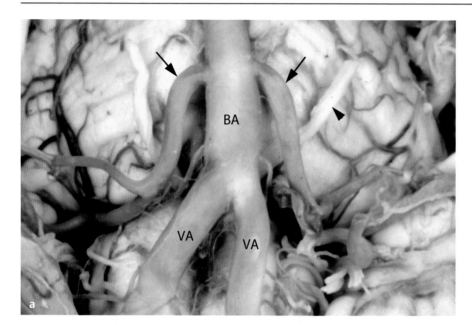

**Fig. 9.16** **(a)** Ventral view of pons and medulla. A dominant anterior inferior cerebellar artery (*upper arrows*).

VA   vertebral artery
BA   basilar artery
Arrowhead   sixth nerve

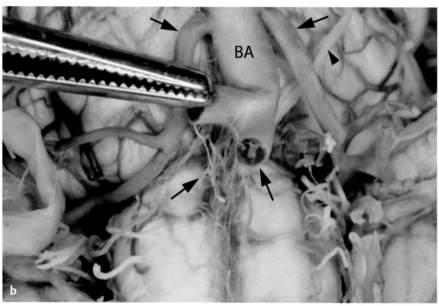

**Fig. 9.16** **(b)** Same specimen as **(a)**. Perforators (*left lower arrow*) to medulla from the posterior vertebro-basilar junction.

Upper arrows   anterior inferior
                 cerebellar arteries
Right lower arrow   vertebral artery
BA   basilar artery
Arrowhead   sixth nerve

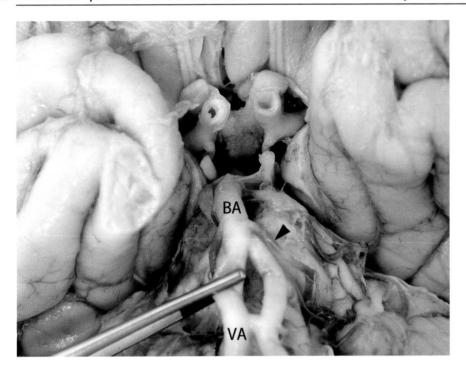

**Fig. 9.17** Fenestration of the basilar artery in its lower third.

BA  basilar artery
VA  vertebral artery
Arrowhead   anterior inferior
                 cerebellar artery

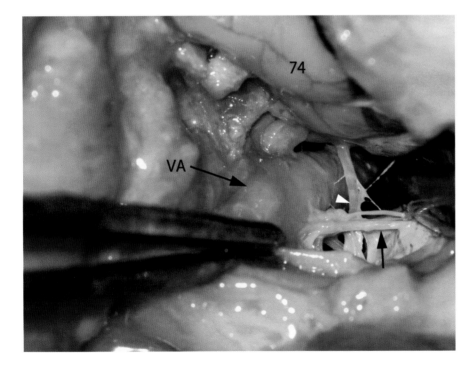

**Fig. 9.18** Suboccipital and left high cervical laminectomy exposing the vertebral artery as it enters the posterior fossa.

VA  vertebral artery
74  cerebellum
Lower arrow   posterior root of C1
                 passing posterior to the
                 spinal accessory nerve
                 (*arrowhead*)

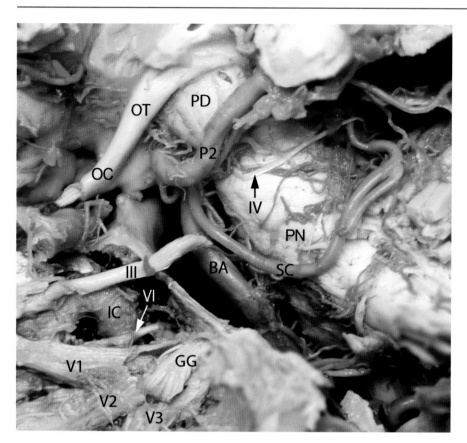

**Fig. 9.19** Lateral view of the left side of the brain stem.

PD   peduncle
OT   optic tract
OC   optic chiasm
P2   posterior cerebral artery
IV   fourth nerve
PN   pons
III   thirrd nerve
SC   superior cerebellar artery
BA   basilar artery
IC   internal carotid artery
VI   sixth nerve
V1   first division of the fifth nerve
V2   second division of the fifth nerve
V3   third division of the fifth nerve
GG   gasserian ganglion

## 9.6 Clinical Cases

### 9.6.1 Case 1

A young woman was referred after discovery of a giant distal vertebral aneurysm during workup for headaches and quadriparesis. A giant, partially thrombosed aneurysm was discovered affecting the distal intracranial vertebral artery with a pouch leading to the origin of a large combined anterior inferior cerebellar artery–posterior inferior cerebellar artery (AICA-PICA) branch. This was treated through jail-ing a microcatheter and using two overlapping flow diverters to cover the neck. Thereafter, the aneurysm was coiled, leaving a single covered pouch leading to a dominant AICA-PICA branch. Follow-up revealed complete remodeling of the vessel and resolution of the patient's symptoms, with preservation of the combined AICA-PICA trunk.

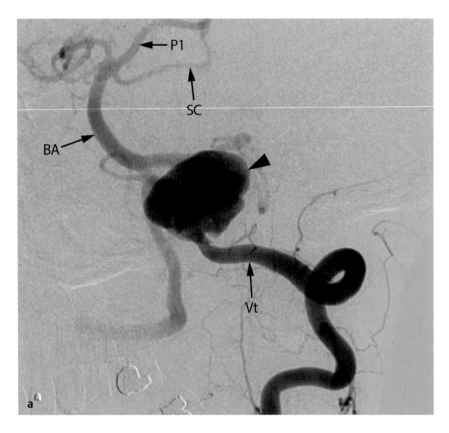

**Fig. 9.20** **(a)** Anteroposterior view of the left vertebral angiogram showing the aneurysm (*arrowhead*).

BA  basilar artery
Vt  vertebral artery
SC  superior cerebral artery
P1  posterior cerebral artery

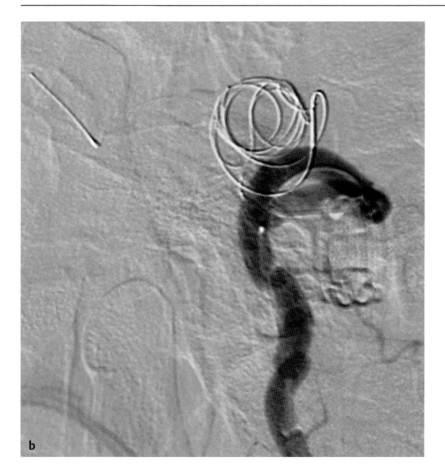

b

**Fig. 9.20** (*Continued*) **(b)** A stent diverter inserted with coils in the aneurysm.

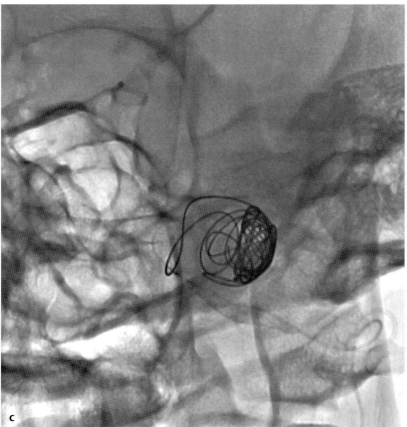

c

**Fig. 9.20** **(c)** More coils are inserted.

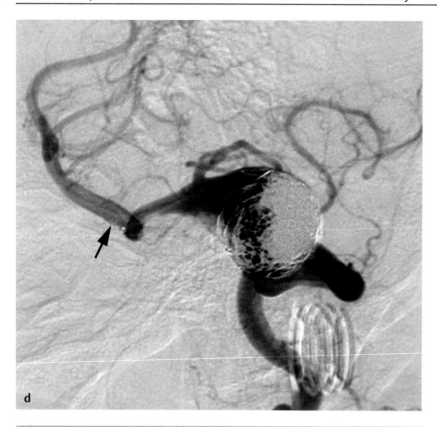

**Fig. 9.20** (*Continued*) **(d)** Three stent-flow diverters have been inserted in the left vertebral artery passing into the basilar artery (*arrow*). More coils have been introduced into the aneurysm.

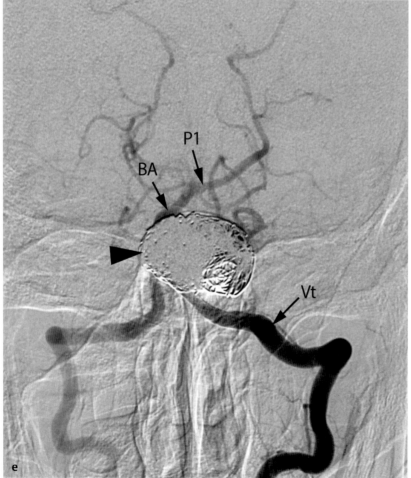

**Fig. 9.20** **(e)** Follow-up left vertebral angiogram showing complete obliteration of the aneurysm (*arrowhead*) and patency of the vertebrobasilar system.

BA   basilar artery
P1   left posterior cerebral artery
Vt   left vertebral artery

## 9.6.2 Case 2

A middle-aged woman was discovered to have an incidental vertebrobasilar junction aneurysm with an associated fenestration of the proximal basilar artery. Given the symmetry of both branches of the fenestration, two braided stents were placed in each trunk, extending from the ipsilateral vertebral artery to the fenestration limb. A microcatheter that had been previously jailed in the aneurysm was used for coiling. The patient made an unremarkable recovery. Follow-up angiography revealed patency of both limbs and occlusion of the aneurysm.

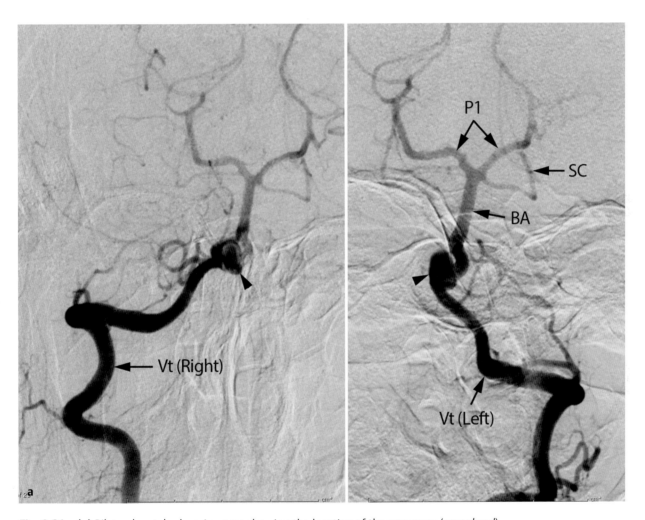

**Fig. 9.21** **(a)** Bilateral vertebral angiograms showing the location of the aneurysm (*arrowhead*).

Vt    vertebral artery
BA    basilar artery
P1    posterior cerebral arteries
SC    superior cerebral artery

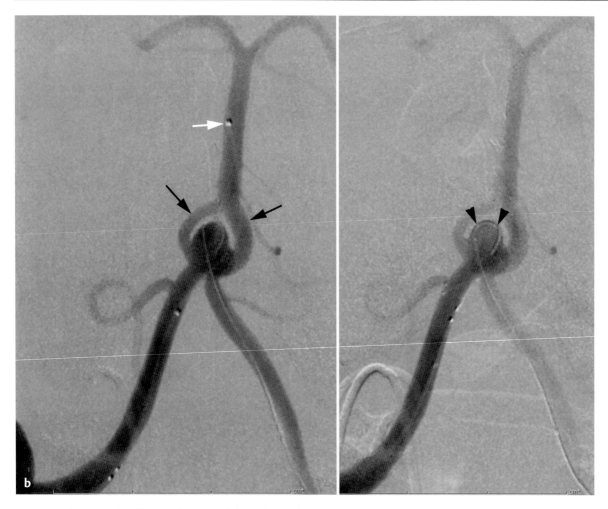

**Fig. 9.21** (*Continued*)   **(b)** Simultaneous bilateral vertebral angiograms. The aneurysm is located in a congenitally fenestrated section of the basilar artery (*lower arrows*). A microcatheter is visible in the basilar artery (*upper arrow*) and a microcatheter is seen inside the aneurysm (*double arrowheads*).

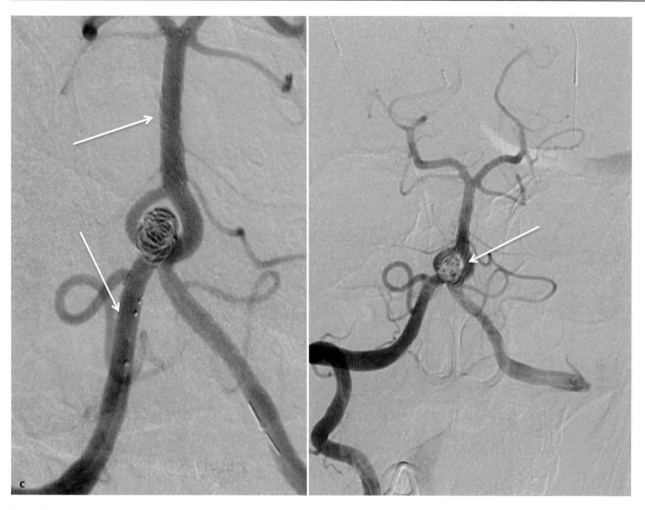

**Fig. 9.21** (*Continued*)   **(c)** A stent is deployed via the right vertebral artery (*left lower arrow*) into the basilar artery (*left upper arrow*). There is further coiling of the aneurysm (*right arrow*).

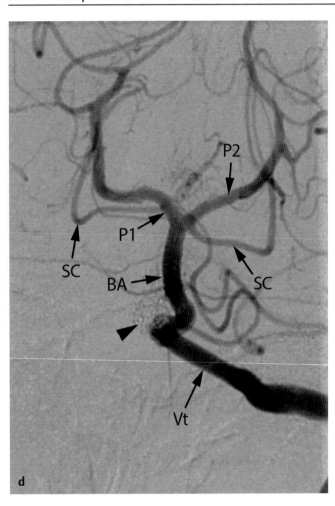

**Fig. 9.21** (*Continued*) **(d)** Left vertebral angiogram at 6-month follow-up shows complete obliteration of the aneurysm (*arrowhead*).

P1, P2  posterior cerebral artery
SC       superior cerebellar artery
Vt       left vertebral artery
BA       basilar artery

### 9.6.3 Case 3

A 42-year-old man presented with a cerebellar hemorrhage and dysmetria. The workup, including magnetic resonance imaging, revealed a large, almost hemispheric, arteriovenous malformation (AVM) fed from all three major branches of the basilar system, namely, the superior cerebellar artery (SCA), anterior inferior cerebellar artery (AICA), and posterior inferior cerebellar artery (PICA). This was treated through staged embolization with a liquid embolic agent. Minimal residual filling of the AVM through small terminal branches of the SCA, AICA, and PICA was noted. These were considered too small to catheterize and, given the original large size, surgery was not considered further. The patient was therefore treated with gamma knife radiosurgery. At 2-year follow-up, the AVM had completely disappeared, and the patient made an excellent recovery and returned to work.

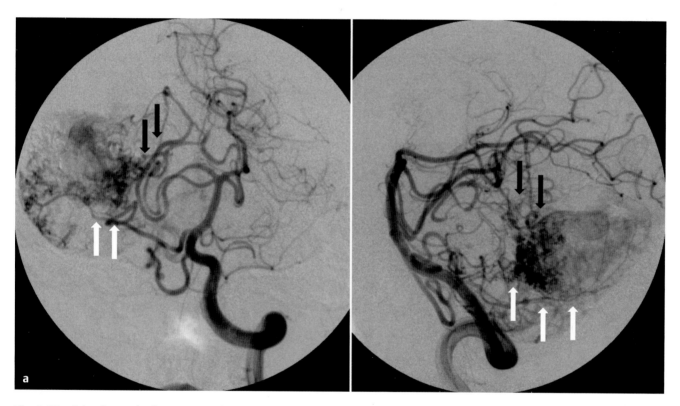

**Fig. 9.22  (a)** Left vertebral angiogram shows an arteriovenous malformation with contributions from the right superior cerebellar artery (*upper arrows*) and the right anterior inferior cerebellar artery (*lower arrows*).

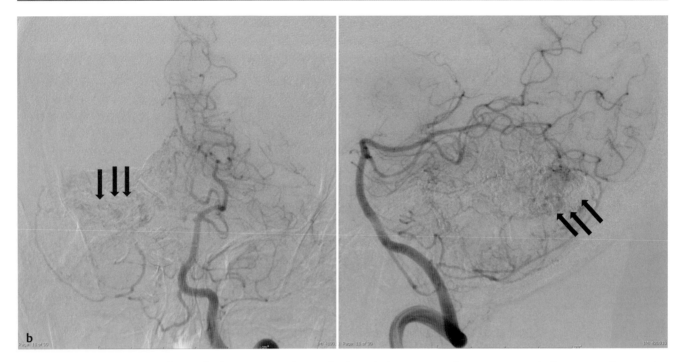

**Fig. 9.22** (*Continued*)   **(b)** Left vertebral angiogram after multiple embolizations via the superior cerebellar artery, the anterior inferior cerebellar artery, and the posterior inferior cerebellar artery. There is still some residual filling of the arteriovenous malformation (*arrows*).

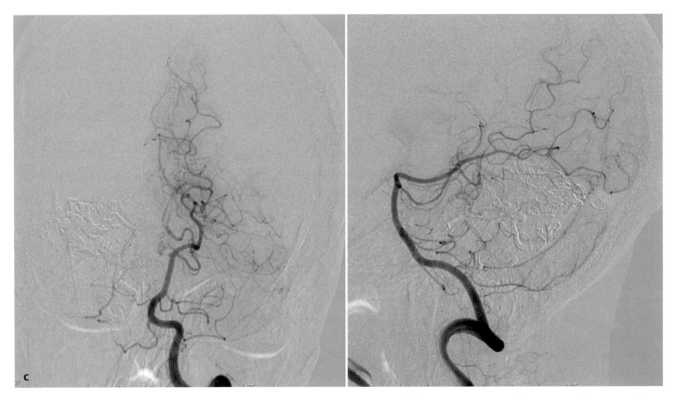

**Fig. 9.22**   **(c)** Left vertebral angiogram 2 years after gamma knife treatment of the arteriovenous malformation. There is no filling of the arteriovenous malformation.

## Clinical Pearls

- Anastomoses between the vertebral artery over the C1 arch and occipital artery branches are the rule rather than the exception. In cases of atherosclerotic occlusion of the dominant vertebral artery, the occipital anastomoses may be the primary supply to the posterior circulation. These connections can be robust enough to give the semblance of the proatlantal variant of primitive fetal anastomoses between the carotid and vertebral arteries.

  During embolization of occipital artery feeders to dural arteriovenous fistulas, particularly at the transverse sigmoid junction, these anastomoses, which may not be overtly evident on angiography, are especially dangerous.

- Upon opening of the dura, the vertebral entry into the subarachnoid space is typically located below the first dentate ligament and the spinal branch of the accessory nerve.

### Posterior Inferior Cerebellar Artery

- The posterior inferior cerebellar artery (PICA) also provides branches in its tonsillar segment to the posterior cord in the form of posterior spinal arteries.

- Occlusion of the PICA presents frequently with Wallenberg's syndrome, affecting the ipsilateral face and contralateral body sensation, along with ipsilateral dysmetria resulting from effects on the inferior cerebellar peduncle, nausea and omiting from effects on the reticular formation, and area postrema. These deficits typically resolve.

- The two tonsillar loops of the PICA are in close proximity to each other in the midline and ideally situated for a PICA-PICA bypass for intended or observed occlusion of one PICA.

- PICA aneurysms are typically very broad based and, based on close proximity to the entry of the vertebral artery, are ideally treated by being clipped through a far lateral skull-base approach. During clipping, it is key to be able to separate the fibers of the vagus and glossopharyngeal nerves, which overlie the PICA and its origin, from excessive manipulation and entrapment by the clip.

### Anterior Spinal Artery

- Anterior spinal arteries are frequently paired; however, it is important to identify them when planning to deconstruct a terminal vertebral artery segment during intervention for dissections or aneurysms, because this may result in occlusion of the dominant spinal artery with resultant quadriplegia.

### Vertebrobasilar Junction

- The vertebrobasilar junction is quite frequently populated on its ventral surface by perforators to the medulla. This is a frequent site for large and giant vertebrobasilar aneurysms and aneurysms related to fenestrations in the proximal basilar artery. Aneurysms in this location can be approached through a far lateral skull-base approach.

### Anterior Inferior Cerebellar Artery

- The anterior inferior cerebellar artery (AICA) frequently communicates with terminal petrosal branches of the middle meningeal artery, as well as the neuromeningeal branch of the ascending pharyngeal artery. Aneurysms in this location are rare and best treated endovascularly. Open approaches are complicated and include a traditional retrosigmoid approach, as well as skull-base approaches through a presigmoid corridor, as well as the middle fossa Kawase approach, which requires drilling of the petrous apex. The AICA is a frequent offender during microvascular decompression for facial tic.

### Superior Cerebellar Artery

- The SCA is typically superficially located in the tentorial incisura and can be used as a recipient for a superficial temporal to SCA bypass for basilar ischemia or flow reversal during treatment of aneurysms.

- The SCA is frequently involved in pial dural arteriovenous fistulas draining into tentorial veins secondary to a tentorial branch from the SCA (artery of Davidoff and Schechter), which provides arterial supply to the tentorium. This artery has also been implicated in nonaneurysmal perimesencephalic subarachnoid hemorrhage.

- Although the basilar terminus and P1 segments are crowded by brainstem perforators, the superior cerebellar artery origin is typically devoid of major perforators, which renders a transsylvian exposure for clipping an excellent option.

# 10 Venous Anatomy

## 10.1 Venous Sinuses of the Dura Mater

### 10.1.1 Superior Sagittal Sinus

The superior sagittal sinus starts anteriorly in the margins of the falx at the crista galli and extends posteriorly along a groove in the midline of the skull, usually slightly to the right of the midline. It terminates in the torcular Herophili at the internal occipital protuberance, most often flowing into the right transverse sinus. The superior cerebral veins enter the sinus and, as they terminate, turn anteriorly and enter the superior sagittal sinus against the venous flow. There are no valves in the superior sagittal sinus or in the other venous structures of the brain and dura. The midportion of the superior sagittal sinus is particularly rough along its floor, with folds of dura and irregular entry sites of the venous structures. The floor of the superior sagittal sinus is smoother in the frontal and occipital regions. The arachnoid granulations are particularly prominent in the midportion of the sinus as well. On cross section, the superior sagittal sinus, particularly in its midportion, may be divided by tough dural septa (chordae willisii) into multiple longitudinal compartments. These are usually less evident in the occipital region prior to it entering the torcular Herophili.

### 10.1.2 Inferior Sagittal Sinus

The inferior sagittal sinus is formed in the posterior two-thirds of the free margin of the falx. Its interior is quite smooth, without septa, and of much smaller size than the superior sagittal sinus. It terminates in the vein of Galen. On occasion, one may see a medial cerebral vein of small diameter entering the inferior sagittal sinus.

### 10.1.3 Straight Sinus

The straight sinus is formed at the junction of the falx with the tentorium and extends backward from the point of confluence of the inferior sagittal sinus and the great vein of Galen. In general, the superior cerebellar vein enters the vein of Galen rather than the straight sinus. The straight sinus tends to enter the confluence of a torcular Herophili on the left rather than the right and flows into the left transverse sinus.

### 10.1.4 Transverse Sinus

The transverse sinuses course from medial to lateral in horizontal grooves in the attached margin of the tentorium at the occipital cranium. Each one courses laterally toward the base of the petrous bone. The transverse sinuses then enter the sigmoid sinuses as they extend inferiorly, somewhat anteriorly and medially, to enter the jugular bulb. One transverse sinus and sigmoid sinus may be less developed than their counterparts on the opposite side.

At the junction of the transverse sinus and sigmoid sinus, the superior petrosal sinus invariably enters the confluence of the transverse sinus as it converts to the sigmoid sinus. The occipital sinus, which drains from the posterior edge of the foramen magnum and along the edge of the cerebellar falx, usually terminates in one of the sigmoid sinuses.

Emissary veins pass from the scalp and extracranial soft tissues through foramina and fissures communicating with the transverse and sigmoid sinuses. The mastoid emissary vein passes through a foramen in the skull medial to the mastoid process and connects the transverse sinus with veins of the soft tissues of the occipital region. The condyloid emissary vein passes through the condyloid foramen superior to the condyles at the base of the cranium and connects the periarterial extradural venous structures surrounding the vertebral artery with the lower portion of the sigmoid sinus. A venous plexus or vein can accompany the hypoglossal nerve through its foramen connecting to the occipital sinus and veins of the medulla.

### 10.1.5 Superior Petrosal Sinus

Each superior petrosal sinus is on the superior border of the petrous bone attached to the tentorium cerebelli and extends from the cavernous to the transverse sinus, entering at the junction of the transverse sinus and sigmoid sinus. These sinuses have a smooth-walled interior and bridge the roof of Meckel's cave. The petrosal vein, adjacent to the fifth cranial nerve within the posterior fossa, frequently enters the superior petrosal sinus superiorly.

### 10.1.6 Inferior Petrosal Sinus

The paired inferior petrosal sinuses are formed as they exit the posterior cavernous sinus and extend along a suture between the petrous bone and the basisphenoid bone. They are intimately related to the exit of the ninth nerve and may exit joining the jugular bulb in the anterior compartment or extend through a separate foramen into the upper cervical region joining the internal jugular vein separately. Even when the jugular bulb and the ipsilateral internal jugular vein are well undeveloped, the inferior petrosal vein may form a large tributary to the internal jugular vein in the neck. The tenth and eleventh nerves are more intimately related to the medial and anterior wall of the jugular bulb.

### 10.1.7 Sphenoparietal Sinus

The sphenoparietal sinus extends under the inner aspect of the lesser wing of the sphenoid, emptying into the cavernous sinus. It receives branches from the superficial middle cerebral vein, bridging from the anterior temporal lobe to this sinus and subsequently draining into the cavernous sinus.

### 10.1.8 Cavernous Sinus

The cavernous sinus is a paired venous dural structure. Each sinus begins at the medial border of the superior orbital fissure. The sinuses communicate and receive tributaries from the ophthalmic, sphenoparietal, and superficial middle cerebral veins. Within each sinus and its dural walls are located the internal carotid artery; the third, fourth, and sixth nerves; and the first division of the fifth nerve.

The circular sinus is formed by a circular venous cavity in a dural leaf on the edges of the diaphragma sellae anterior and posterior to the pituitary body, forming a connection between the two cavernous sinuses. The anterior aspect of the circular sinus is usually larger.

The basilar venous plexus lies along the clivus and connects the posterior cavernous sinus with the inferior petrosal sinuses. Posteriorly, the cavernous sinus communicates with the superior petrosal sinus.

The superior ophthalmic vein courses posteriorly with the ophthalmic artery in the orbit and runs superiorly through the superior orbital fissure external to the annulus of Zinn. It enters the cavernous sinus between the nasociliary nerve and the sixth nerve just behind the annulus of Zinn at the apex of the orbit. The entry of the superior ophthalmic vein into the cavernous sinus is buried in a dural leaf. Just prior to entry into the cavernous sinus, the inferior ophthalmic vein usually joins the superior ophthalmic vein.

There is an emissary venous plexus surrounding the infratemporal mandibular nerve at the foramen ovale that connects the cavernous sinus with the pterygoid plexus in the infratemporal fossa. The internal carotid venous plexus accompanies the internal carotid artery in the carotid canal connecting the cavernous sinus with parapharyngeal venous plexuses in the neck.

## 10.2 Vein of Galen

The great vein of Galen enters the dural venous structures superior to the pineal gland and around the splenium of the corpus callosum, extending in a curved fashion superiorly and posteriorly to enter the confluence of the straight sinus. The vein of Galen is smooth walled and has multiple tributaries in its short course prior to entering the dural venous cavities. The internal cerebral veins join the vein of Galen, coursing under the splenium of the corpus callosum above the pineal gland from the roof of the third ventricle. Superiorly, the veins of the corpus callosum drain either into the junction of the internal cerebral vein or directly into the vein of Galen. There are inferior cerebral veins that drain the medial parietal-occipital region, which drain directly into the vein of Galen. Bilaterally, the basal veins of Rosenthal also join the vein of Galen, as well as the superior cerebellar vein. All the branches of the vein of Galen enter a common compartment in its proximal portion, and, thereafter, a singular **J**-shaped vein drains into the straight sinus.

## 10.3 Deep Veins and Cortical Tributaries

### 10.3.1 Basal Vein of Rosenthal

The basal vein of Rosenthal begins at the anterior perforated substance at the base of the brain. It is initially formed by the confluence of the deep middle cerebral vein and veins draining from the suprachiasmatic region and from the region of the mammillary bodies. It receives tributaries from the medial temporal lobe and brainstem, but in particular, receives at times a large vein draining the choroid plexus of the temporal horn.

### 10.3.2 Internal Cerebral Veins

The two internal cerebral veins are formed by the confluence of each thalamostriate vein in the lateral ventricle, the large serpentine choroid vein, and the anterior septal vein running in the septum pellucidum. Each internal cerebral vein is located in the roof of the third ventricle between the arachnoid layers of the velum interpositum, but usually more intimately adherent to the inferior layer. Each internal cerebral vein courses posteriorly in the midline to enter on either side of the vein of Galen. In the roof of the third ventricle, the internal cerebral veins are intimately associated with the tela choroidea.

The tela choroidea consists of two pial membranous layers in the roof of the third ventricle. If the two layers are separated, they form the cistern of the velum interpositum. The upper pial membrane is attached to the undersurface of the fornix. The lower membrane is attached to the taenia choroidea (thalami), the stria medullaris (thalami), and the pineal body. The thalamostriate vein runs forward in the floor of the lateral ventricle in a groove between the caudate nucleus and the thalamus. It terminates at the apex of the tela choroidea where it is joined by the anterior septal vein and the vein of the choroid plexus to form the internal cerebral vein in the roof of the third ventricle. This confluence is somewhat obscured by the choroid plexus lying over the posterior-inferior margin of the foramen of Monro. The entry of the thalamostriate vein into the internal cerebral vein at the foramen of Monro can vary. It can pierce the anterior thalamus and enter the third ventricle in the midportion or penetrate the septum pellucidum posterior to the foramen of Monro to join the internal cerebral vein. The thalamostriate vein can also be deep to the subependymal layer and not clearly visible on the floor of the lateral ventricle.

### 10.3.3 Superficial Cerebral Veins

There are twelve or more superior cerebral veins, which are located superior and lateral on the surface of the cerebral hemisphere. They run upward to the interhemispheric fissure and receive tributaries from the medial hemisphere. The superior cerebral veins terminate in the superior sagittal sinus or in the lateral lacunae (venous lakes) of the superior sagittal sinus. Their termination is oriented anteriorly and against the flow of the sagittal sinus.

The most prominent superficial cerebral veins are the great vein of Trolard, the vein of Labbé, and the superficial middle cerebral vein. There may be a confluence between the great vein of Trolard, the superficial middle cerebral vein, and the vein of Labbé. The vein of Labbé courses over the posterior temporal region and can traverse a small portion of the tentorium before entering the transverse sinus. The vein of Labbé may originate deep within a sulcus in the posterior temporal lobe and not anastomose with the superficial middle cerebral vein. For this reason, the vein of Labbé may be hard to recognize in its course over the surface of the brain, only to surface just prior to bridging the gap between the brain and the sigmoid–transverse junction.

The superficial middle cerebral vein courses over the superior temporal gyrus extending over the anterior temporal lobe. The insula has a variable venous drainage that may include drainage into the superficial system, as well as the deep venous system. There is a tendency for the posterior insula to drain more frequently into the deep system, whereas the anterior portion of the insula tends to drain into the superficial venous system.

The inferior cerebral hemispheres along the inferior occipital and posterior temporal region may have draining veins that course through the leaves of the dura of the tentorium, entering venous lakes, and then draining into the transverse sinus. In addition, veins from the superior cerebellum can bridge to the inferior surface of the tentorium and then subsequently drain through venous lakes into the transverse sinus.

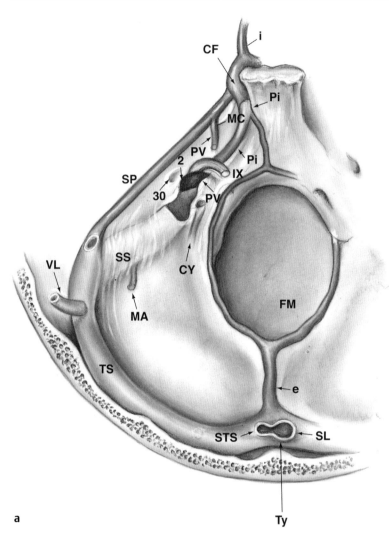

a

**Fig. 10.1 (a)** Superior view into the posterior fossa of the skull, showing the relationships of the venous sinuses.

i     circular sinus of the pituitary fossa
CF   posterior cavernous sinus
MC  Meckel's cave
Pi    inferior petrosal sinus
SP   superior petrosal sinus
PV   petrosal vein
 2    jugular bulb
IX    ninth nerve
30   internal auditory meatus
SS   sigmoid sinus
VL   vein of Labbé
MA  mastoid emissary vein
CY   condyloid emissary vein
FM  foramen magnum
e     midline occipital sinus
SL   sagittal sinus (superior)
STS  straight sinus
TS   transverse sinus
Ty   torcular Herophili (confluence of sinuses)

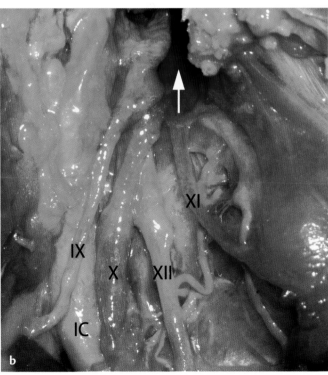

b

**Fig. 10.1 (b)** View of cranial nerves on left side exiting the jugular foramen (*arrow*) medially, with the internal jugular vein removed. Nerve IX passes over and lateral to the internal carotid artery (IC). The hypoglossal nerve (XII) is seen descending deep to IX, X, XI and then to pass more superficial and over the external carotid artery (*not shown*).

XI   eleventh nerve
X    tenth nerve
IX   ninth nerve

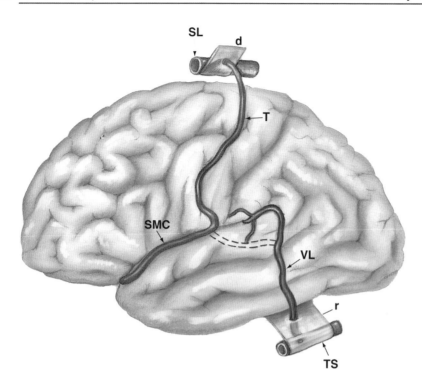

**Fig. 10.2** Lateral view of the left cerebral hemisphere indicating the relationships between the superficial middle cerebral vein, great vein of Trolard, and the vein of Labbé.

| | |
|---|---|
| d | dura |
| r | dura of tentorium |
| SMC | superficial middle cerebral vein |
| SL | sagittal sinus (superior) |
| T | great vein of Trolard |
| TS | transverse sinus |
| VL | vein of Labbé |

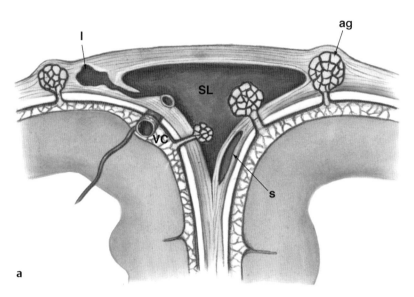

**Fig. 10.3** **(a)** Coronal view at the midsuperior sagittal sinus.

ag arachnoid granulations
l venous lake
s sagittal sinus pocket
SL sagittal sinus (superior)
VC draining cortical vein

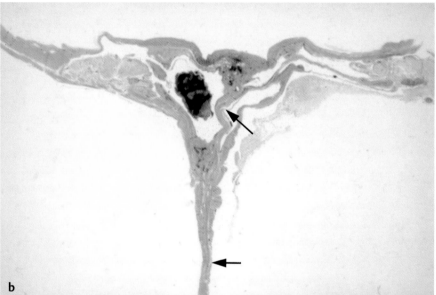

**Fig. 10.3** **(b)** Cross section through the midsuperior sagittal sinus, showing the internal septum (*upper arrow*) dividing the sinus into two compartments.

Lower arrow falx cerebri

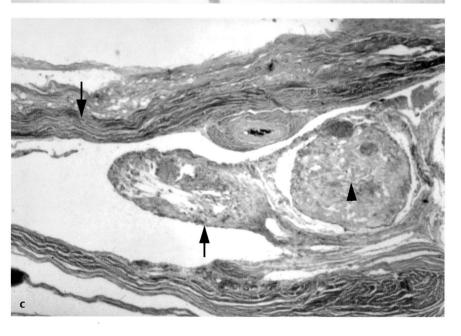

**Fig. 10.3** **(c)** A cross section of a dural leaf, lateral to the superior sagittal sinus, showing a venous lake with arachnoid granulation (*lower right arrow and arrowhead*) protruding into it. External dura continuous with the roof of the superior sagittal sinus is shown (*upper left arrow*).

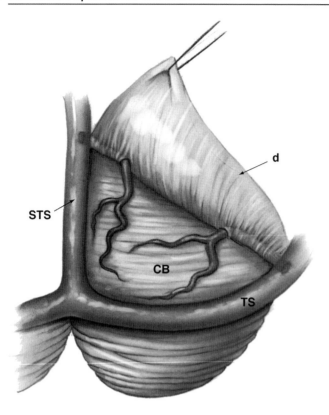

**Fig. 10.4** The tentorium overlying the cerebellum is elevated to show the cerebellar veins over its superior surface draining into the straight sinus and transverse sinus via venous lakes and tunneling in the dura of the tentorium.

d    dura
CB   cerebellum
TS   transverse sinus
STS  straight sinus

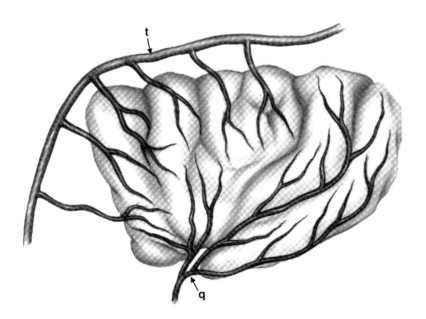

**Fig. 10.5** Lateral view of the left insular region, showing the venous drainage pattern. The insular region has variable venous drainage into the deep and superficial systems.

t    superficial middle cerebral system
q    deep venous drainage system

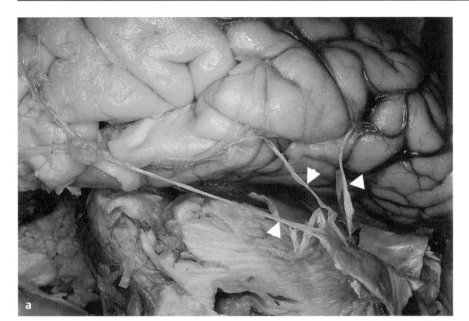

**Fig. 10.6   (a)** Lateral view of the left occipital-temporal lobe. The vein of Labbé (*lower left arrowhead*) is coursing from the posterior temporal lobe to the dura of the tentorium before entering the transverse sinus. Other inferior draining veins from the occipital-temporal region going into venous lakes in the tentorium are shown (*two upper arrowheads*). These other veins should be distinguished from the true vein of Labbé.

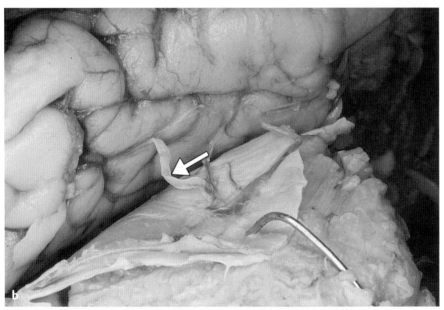

**Fig. 10.6   (b)** Arrow indicates a single inferior occipital-temporal vein draining into a venous lake in the roof of the tentorium.

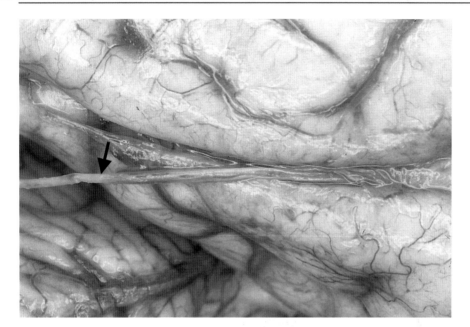

**Fig. 10.7** Lateral view of posterior temporal cerebral hemisphere on the right, showing the emergence of the vein of Labbé (*arrow*) from the depths of the sulcus coursing posteriorly toward the transverse sinus (*not shown*).

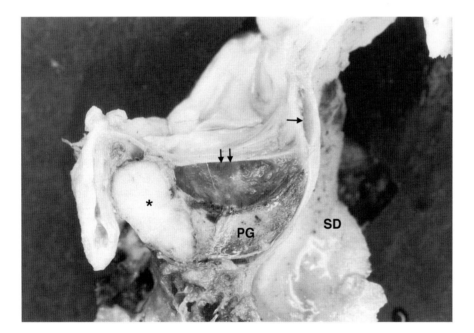

**Fig. 10.8** Medial view of the pituitary gland in sagittal section. Single upper right arrow shows the lumen of the circular sinus. Double small arrows indicate the diaphragma sella above the pituitary gland.

PG    pituitary gland
SD    sphenoid sinus
*       posterior pituitary gland

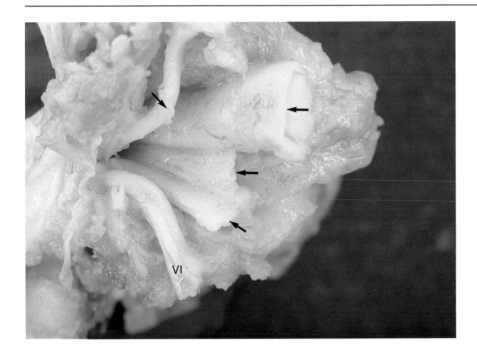

**Fig. 10.9** A lateral anterior view of the apex of the right orbit. Superior division of the third nerve (*upper left arrow*). The inferior division of the third nerve (*lower right arrow*). Optic nerve with dural sheath (*upper right arrow*). Ophthalmic artery (*middle arrow on right*).

VI    sixth nerve

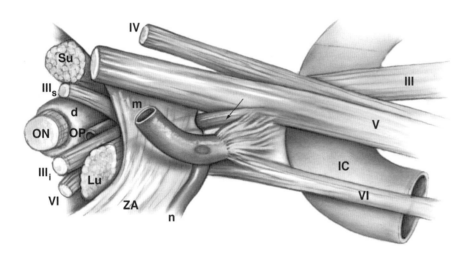

**Fig. 10.10** A lateral view of the apex of the orbit at the annulus of Zinn on the left side, showing the relationship of the cranial nerves at the anterior cavernous sinus and the cranial nerves entering the apex of the orbit. Note that the superior ophthalmic vein courses into the anterior cavernous sinus above the sixth nerve and below the first division of the fifth nerve and is exterior to the annulus of Zinn. The only portion of the first division of the fifth nerve that goes within the annulus of Zinn is the nasocilliary nerve (*arrow*).

IC    internal carotid artery
III    third nerve
III$_s$    superior division of third nerve
III$_i$    inferior division of third nerve
V    first division of the fifth nerve
IV    fourth nerve
n    inferior ophthalmic vein
m    superior ophthalmic vein
ZA    annulus of Zinn
Lu    lateral rectus muscle
OP    ophthalmic artery
Su    superior rectus muscle
d    dura over optic nerve
ON    optic nerve
VI    sixth nerve

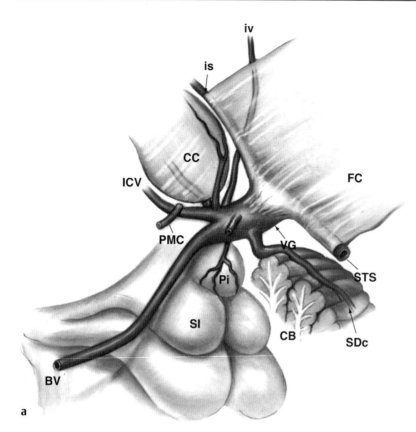

a

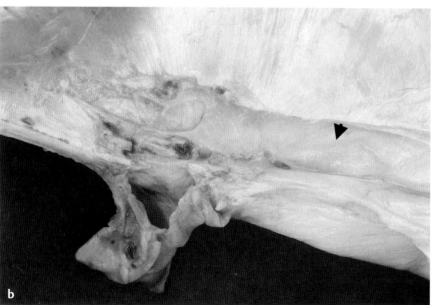

b

**Fig. 10.11** **(a)** A posterior and lateral view of the vein of Galen from the left side.

| | |
|---|---|
| is | inferior sagittal sinus |
| iv | inferior cerebral vein |
| CC | corpus collosum |
| FC | falx |
| STS | straight sinus |
| VG | vein of Galen |
| PMC | posterior medial choroidal artery |
| ICV | internal cerebral vein |
| CB | cerebellum |
| SDc | superior cerebellar vein |
| SI | superior colliculus |
| BV | basal vein of Rosenthal |
| Pi | pineal |

**Fig. 10.11** **(b)** A lateral view of inferior falx showing the entry of the vein of Galen (*lower left arrow*) into the straight sinus (*arrowhead*). As the vein of Galen enters the straight sinus, it is encased in a tougher dural sheath.

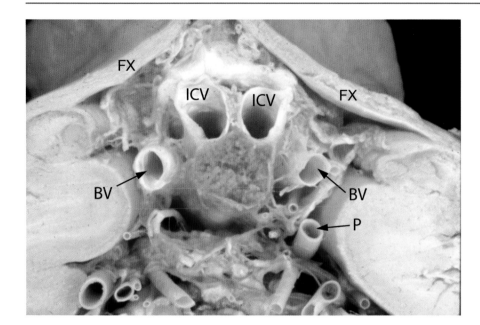

**Fig. 10.12** Coronal section through the posterior fornix region in the area just prior to the entry of the internal cerebral veins into the vein of Galen. A section of the pineal gland can be seen just below the two internal cerebral veins.

BV    basal vein of Rosenthal
FX    fornix
ICV   internal cerebral vein
P      posterior cerebral artery

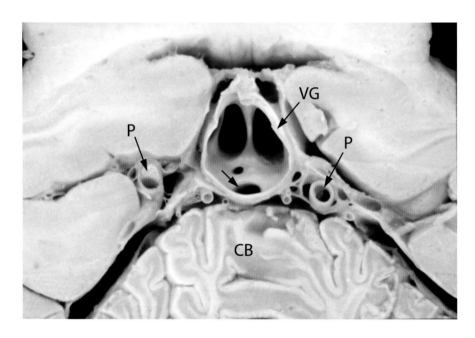

**Fig. 10.13** A coronal section through the vein of Galen posteriorly at the level of the splenium of the corpus collosum. This is just prior to the vein of Galen turning superiorly to enter the straight sinus. Arrow indicates the entrance of the superior cerebellar vein. Note the septum dividing the vein of Galen on either side of which is entering the appropriate internal cerebral vein.

CB    cerebellum
P      posterior cerebral artery
VG    vein of Galen

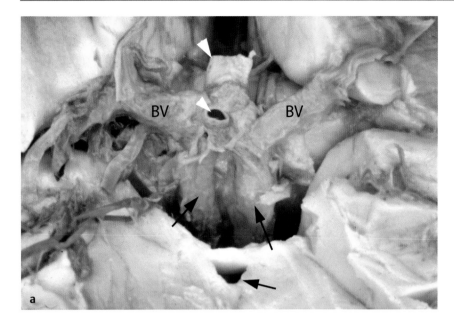

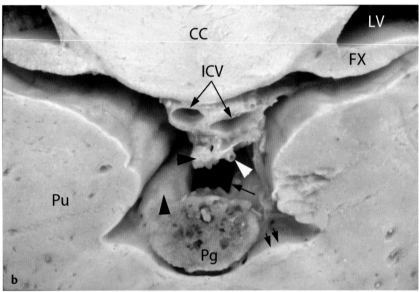

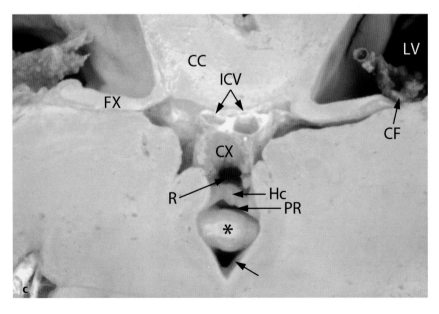

**Fig. 10.14** **(a)** Posterior view at the confluens at the vein of Galen (*upper arrowhead*).

BV   basal vein of Rosenthal
Two opposing arrows   internal cerebral veins
Lower arrow           aqueduct
Lower arrowhead   orifice of entry of superior cerebellar vein into vein of Galen (upper arrowhead)

**Fig. 10.14** **(b)** Coronal section through the level of the midpineal gland (Pg) and viewing anterior.

Arrow   third ventricle
Left upper arrowhead   choroid plexus
ICV  internal cerebral vein
Right arrowhead   branch of the posterior medial choroidal artery
FX   fornix
Pu   pulvinar
Left lower arrowhead   stria medullaris
Lower right arrowheads   trigonis habenulae
LV   lateral ventricle
CC   corpus callosum with beginning of forniceal decussation

**Fig. 10.14** **(c)** Coronal section just anterior to the posterior commissure and looking into the back of the third ventricle.

Lower arrow   aqueduct
*          posterior commissure
PR   pineal recess
Hc   habenular commissure
R    suprapineal recess
CX   choroid plexus
CC   corpus callosum
ICV  internal cerebral veins
FX   fornix
CF   choroidal fissure
LV   lateral ventricle

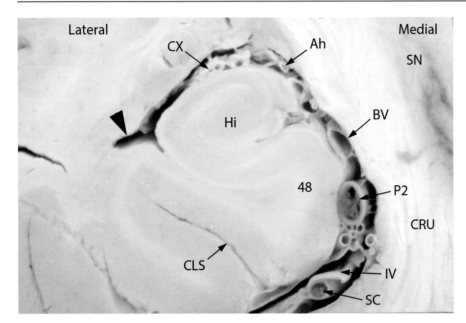

**Fig. 10.15** Cross section through midtemporal lobe.

Arrowhead     ventricle (temporal horn)
Ah     anterior choroidal artery
P2     posterior cerebral artery
SC     superior cerebellar artery
IV     fourth nerve
BV     basal vein of Rosenthal
Hi     hippocampus
48     parahippocampus
CLS     collateral fissure
CRU     crus cerebri
SN     substancia nigra
CX     choroid plexus

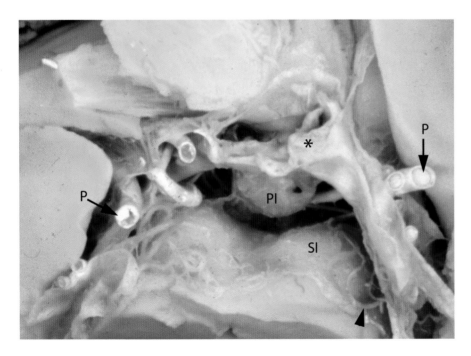

**Fig. 10.16** A posterior view into the quadrigeminal cistern.

SI     superior colliculus
*     arachnoid membrane with vasculature imbedded
Right lower arrowhead     branch of posterior cerebral artery to the superior colliculus
P     posterior cerebral artery
PI     pineal gland

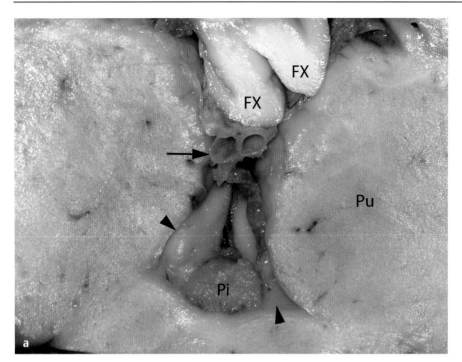

**Fig. 10.17 (a)** Coronal section through the posterior third ventricle and pulvinar (Pu).

Left arrowhead    stria medullaris
Right arrowhead  trigonae habenularis
Pi    pineal gland
FX    fornix
Upper arrow    internal cerebral veins

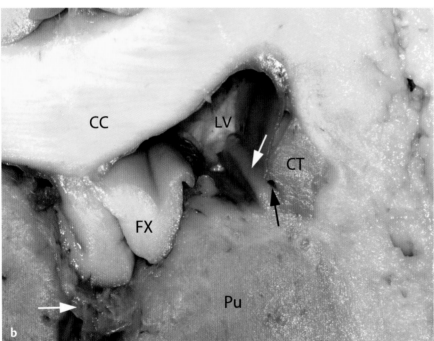

**Fig. 10.17 (b)** Same cross section as **(a)**, looking into lateral ventricle (LV).

CT    caudate nucleus (body)
FX    fornix
Right white arrow   stria terminalis
Black arrow   vena terminalis
Left white arrow    roof of third
                    ventricle with
                    internal cerebral
                    veins
CC    corpus callosum
Pu    pulvinar

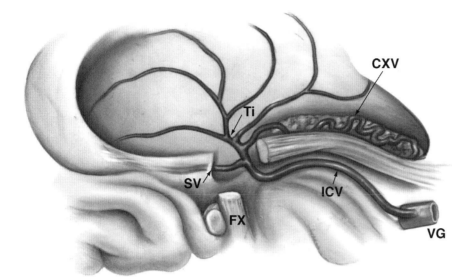

**Fig. 10.18** Medial view of the right internal cerebral vein system. Sagittal view of the right cerebral hemisphere.

CXV   choroid vein
FX    fornix
ICV   internal cerebral vein
SV    anterior septal vein
Ti    thalamostriate vein
VG    vein of Galen

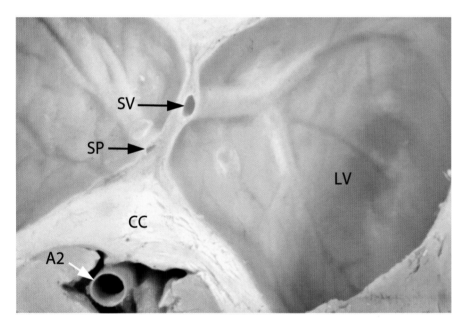

**Fig. 10.19** Viewing from posterior to anterior into frontal horns of lateral ventricles.

SV   anterior septal vein
CC   rostrum of corpus callosum
LV   frontal horn of lateral ventricle
A2   anterior cerebral arteries
SP   septum pellucidum

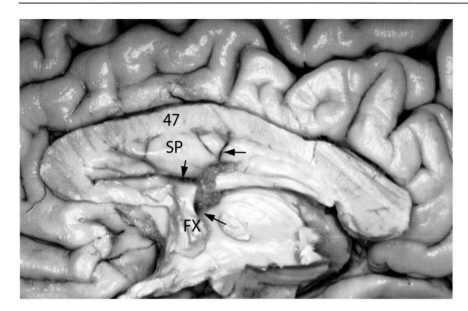

**Fig. 10.20** Sagittal section of right hemisphere (medial view). To left is anterior.

Left arrow     anterior septal vein
Right upper arrow     posterior septal vein
Lower right arrow     foramen of Monro
FX   fornix (pillar)
47   corpus callosum
SP   septum pellucidum

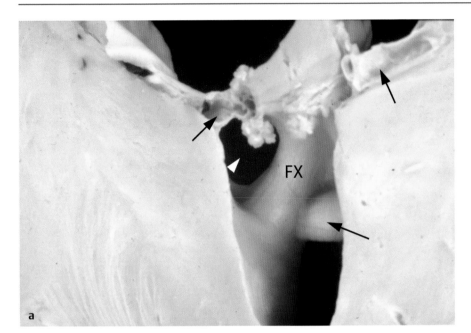

**Fig. 10.21 (a)** A coronal section through the third ventricle viewed from posterior and looking anterior through foramen of Monro on left (*arrowhead*). The thalamostriate veins can be seen draining toward the roof of the third ventricle (*upper arrows on either side*). The anterior commissure (*lower arrow*) is evident, abutting the base of the pillar of the fornix (FX).

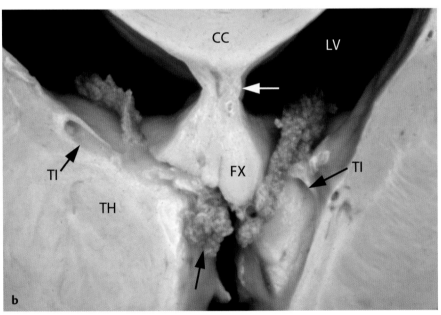

**Fig. 10.21 (b)** Coronal section at the level of the foramen of Monro on both sides and looking posterior.

Black arrow    choroid plexus in third ventricle
FX    body of fornix
CC    corpus callosum
White arrow    septum pellucidum
LV    lateral ventricle
TI    thalamostriate veins entering the foramen of Monro
TH    thalamus

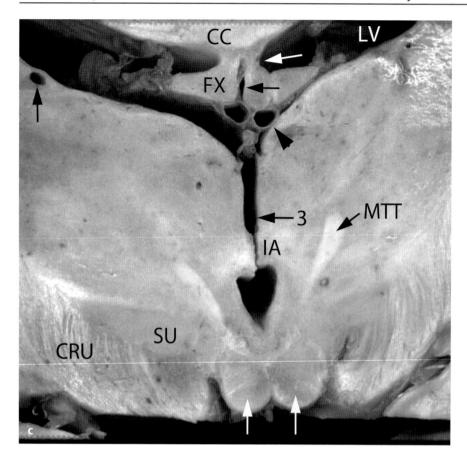

**Fig. 10.21** **(c)** Coronal section at the level of midmammillary bodies (*lower two arrows*). The two internal cerebral veins (*arrowhead*) are in the roof of the third ventricle, with the choroid plexus attached below and fornices (FX) above. Note that the septum pellucidum (*upper horizontal arrow*) becomes thicker and foreshortened as one goes posterior in the body of the lateral ventricle.

CC     corpus callosum
LV     lateral ventricle
3      third ventricle
IA      interthalamic adhesion
CRU   crus cerebri
MTT   mammillothalamic tract
SU     subthalamic nucleus
Lower horizontal arrow   vestigial cistern of the velum interpositum
Upper left arrow   thalamostriate vein

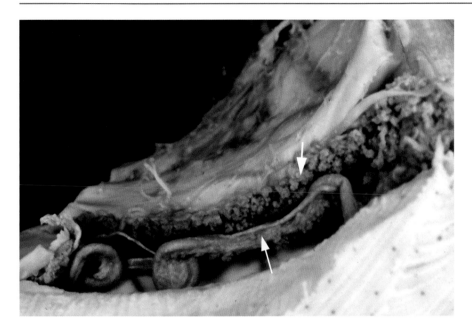

**Fig. 10.22** A section of the brain exposing the lateral ventricular system with the choroid plexus (*upper arrow*) and the tortuous choroid vein (*lower arrow*), which drains into the thalamostriate vein (*not shown*).

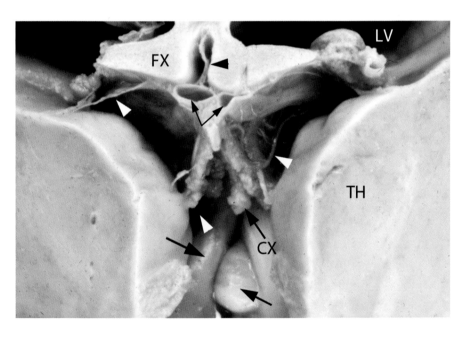

**Fig. 10.23** Coronal section just behind foramen of Monro (*left lower arrowhead*) and viewing from posterior to anterior.

| | |
|---|---|
| Left lower arrow | pillar of fornix |
| Right lower arrow | anterior commissure |
| Upper double arrows | internal cerebral veins imbedded in arachnoid, continuous with the underside of the forniceal arachnoid |
| FX | body of fornix |
| CX | choroid plexus of third ventricle |
| TH | thalamus |
| Top arrowhead | cistern of the velum interpositum |
| LV | lateral ventricle |
| Left arrowhead | arachnoid layer of undersurface of body of fornix, continuous laterally with choroidal fissure |
| Right arrowhead | branch of the posterior medial choroidal artery in the roof of the third ventricle |

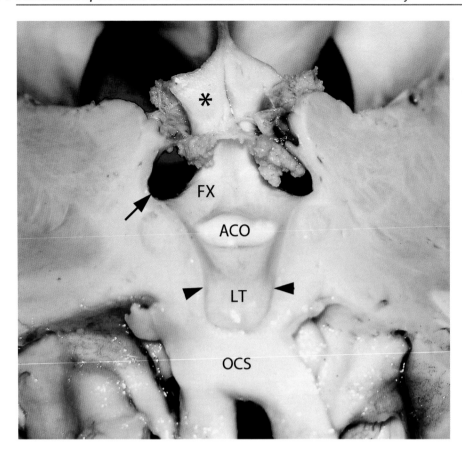

**Fig. 10.24** Coronal section of third ventricle at optic chiasm viewed from posterior to anterior.

FX     pillar of fornix
*       body of fornix
ACO   anterior commissure
OCS   optic chiasm
LT     lamina terminalis
Opposing arrowheads   wall of third
                         ventricle
Arrow   foramen of Monro

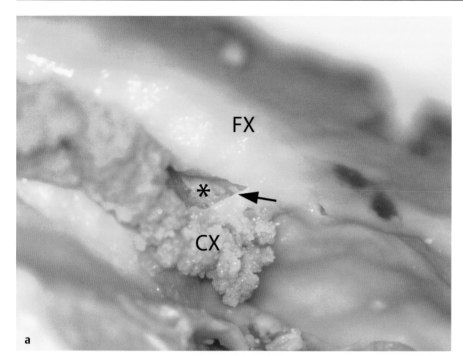

**Fig. 10.25** **(a)** Lateral view into the right lateral ventricle and dissecting open the choroidal fissure (taenia fornis, *arrow*) at its juncture with the fornix (FX) exposing the roof of the third ventricle (*).

CX   choroid plexus

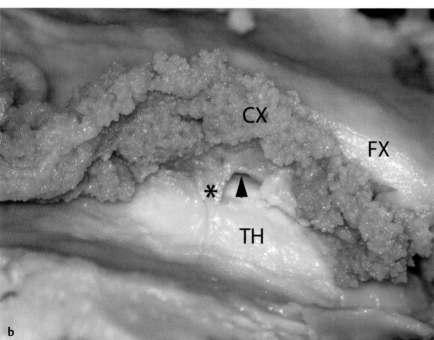

**Fig. 10.25** **(b)** Same specimen as **(a)** except the choroid plexus (CX) is elevated superiorly to open the choroidal fissure (taenia thalami) into the cavity of the third ventricle (*arrowhead*).

TH   thalamus
FX   fornix
*    taenia thalami

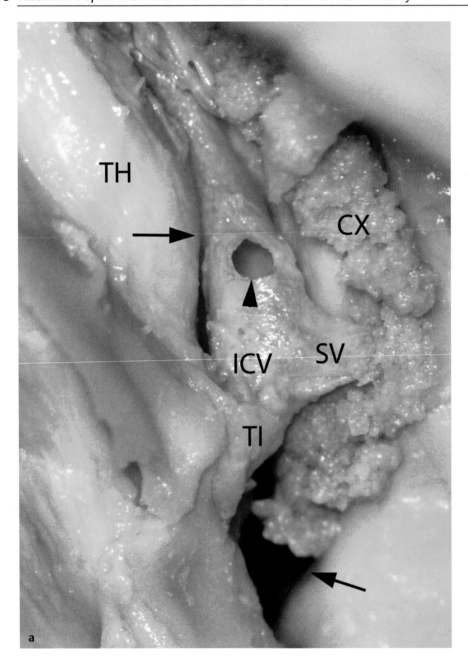

**Fig. 10.26** **(a)** A view into the right lateral ventricle at the foramen of Monro (*right arrow*). The choroid plexus (CX) has been moved medially, opening up the taenia choroidea thalami (*left arrow*) and exposing the roof of the third ventricle.

SV   anterior septal vein
Arrowhead   entry point of choroid vein into internal cerebral vein (ICV)
TH   thalamus
TI   thalamostriate vein that is subependymal entering the ICV

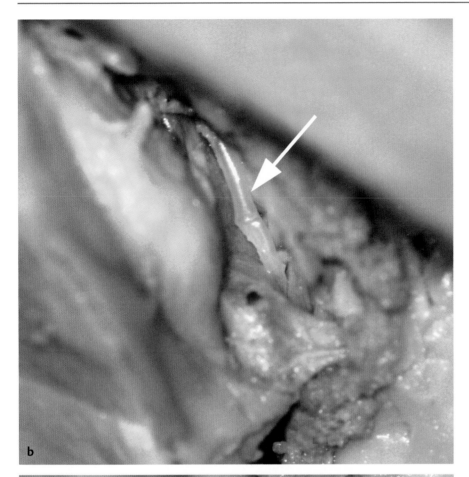

**Fig. 10.26** **(b)** Same specimen as **(a)**. (*Arrow*) A branch of the posterior medial choroidal artery in the roof of the third ventricle overlying the ICV.

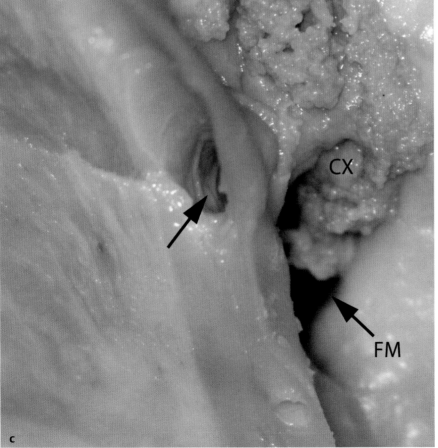

**Fig. 10.26** **(c)** Same specimen as **(a)**. The lumen of the thalamostriate vein (*left arrow*) in its subependymal course to the ICV.

FM  foramen of Monro
CX  choroid plexus

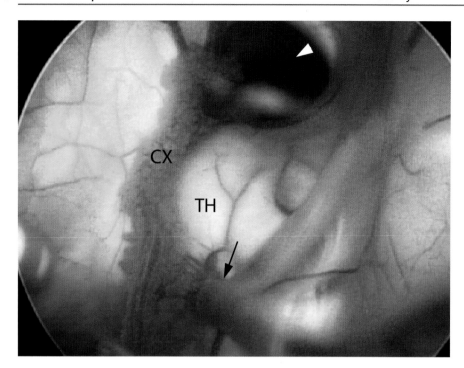

**Fig. 10.27** Endoscopic view into right lateral ventricle. This unusual variation of the thalamostriate vein (*arrow*) terminates into the parenchyma of thalamus well below the foramen of Monro (*arrowhead*).

TH   thalamus
CX   choroid plexus

## 10.4 Clinical Cases

### 10.4.1 Case 1

A 25-year-old woman presented with a history of headaches for many months, but over the last few days had deteriorated and needed ambulance transfer. Initial imaging, including magnetic resonance imaging, suggested bilateral medial infarcts not consistent with arterial territories. Magnetic resonance venography suggested whole sinus infarction. The patient rapidly deteriorated in the emergency room despite anticoagulation. Therefore, the patient was taken to the angiography suite, and transfemoral venous access to the jugular bulb revealed the superior sagittal sinus occlusion. A large-bore aspiration catheter with large stent retrievers was used in the occluded sinus to retrieve the thrombus. Repeat angiography and computed tomography suggested complete resolution of sinus thrombosis. The patient rapidly improved and was discharged home from the hospital on anticoagulation.

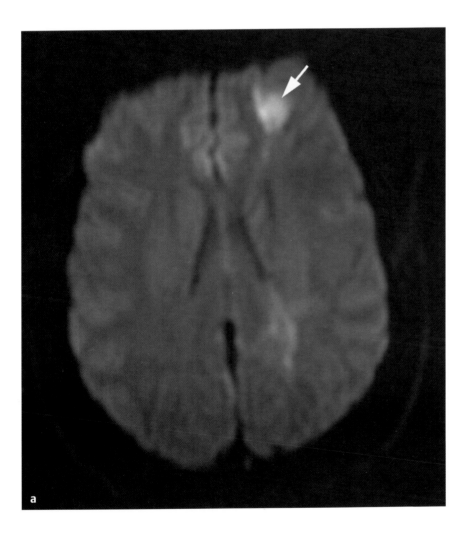

**Fig. 10.28   (a)** Magnetic resonance imaging of the brain indicates an evolving infarct in the left frontal region (*arrow*).

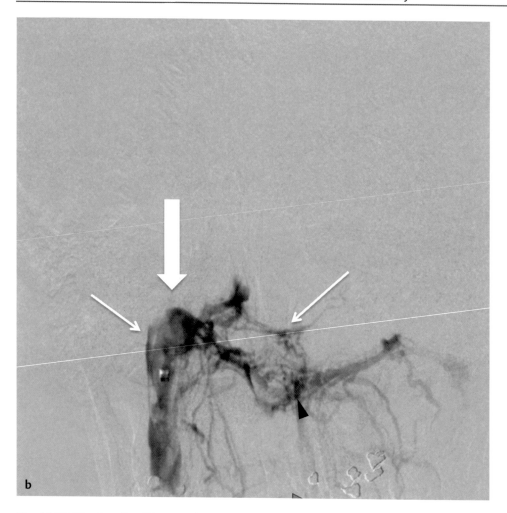

**Fig. 10.28** (*Continued*)    **(b)** A transfemoral venous study of the right internal jugular vein. The transverse sinus does not visualize (*upper arrow*). The jugular bulb (*left arrow*), emissary vein (*right arrow*), and suboccipital venous plexus (*arrowhead*) are shown.

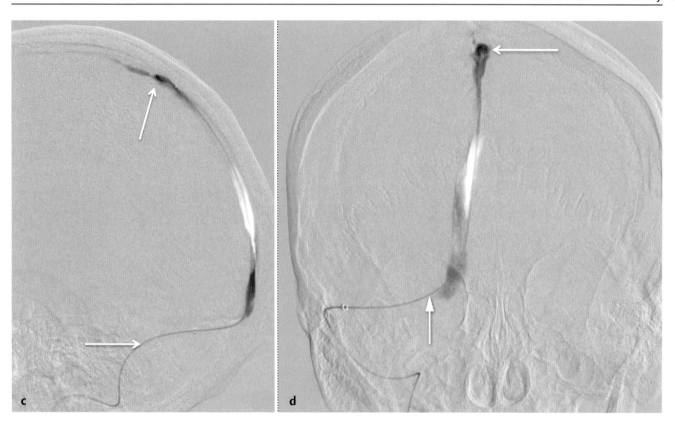

**Fig. 10.28** (*Continued*) **(c)** Lateral view. **(d)** Anteroposterior view shows the catheter in the sigmoid and transverse sinuses (*lower arrow*). Patency of the superior sagittal sinus at the junction of the middle and posterior sections is visible (*upper arrow*).

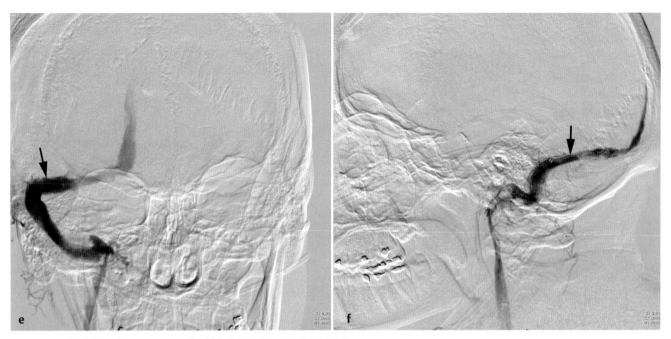

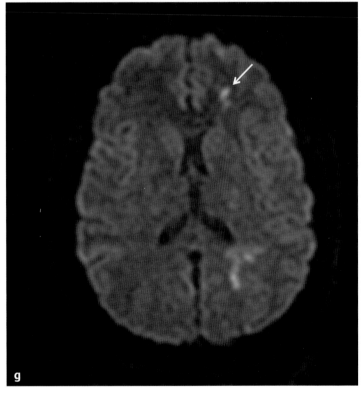

**Fig. 10.28** (*Continued*) **(e)** Anteroposterior view. **(f)** Lateral view. A large-bore aspiration catheter with a large stent retriever was used in the occluded sinus to retrieve the thrombus in the transverse sinus (*arrow*). **(g)** Posttreatment magnetic resonance imaging of the brain shows a marked decrease of the hyperdensity in the left frontal lobe (*arrow*).

## 10.4.2  Case 2

A teenager presented with seizures, and magnetic resonance imaging revealed bilateral midline infarcts. Magnetic resonance venography revealed a sagittal sinus thrombosis. Due to a poor neurological exam, despite systemic heparinization, she was brought to the angiography suite and a microcatheter was placed in the anterior sagittal sinus. Intravenous tissue plasminogen activator was dripped continuously through the sinus with daily angiograms. Over three days she recanalized her sinus with concurrent improvement in the neurological examination.

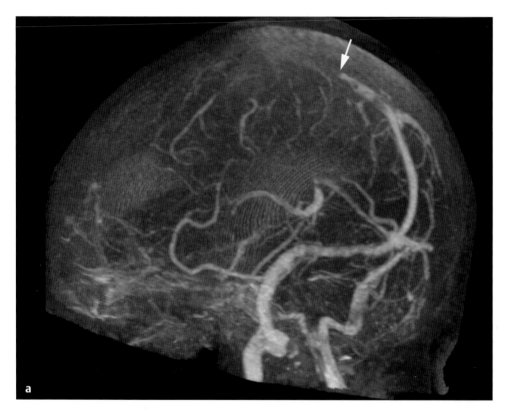

**Fig. 10.29** **(a)** Magnetic resonance venogram shows a superior sinus thrombosis at the junction of the middle and posterior superior sagittal sinus (*arrow*).

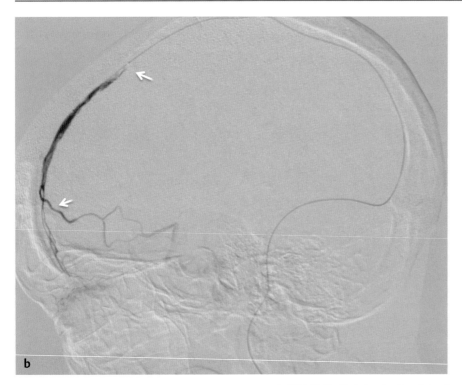

**Fig. 10.29** (*Continued*) **(b)** A microcatheter (*upper arrow*) was inserted in the superior sagittal sinus anteriorly for the tissue plasminogen activator drip. Frontal cortical vein is indicated (*lower arrow*).

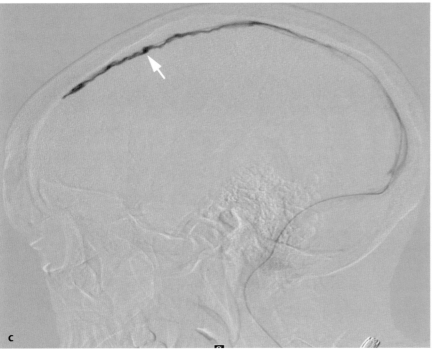

**Fig. 10.29** **(c)** Venogram shows the filling of the anterior superior sagittal sinus (*arrow*).

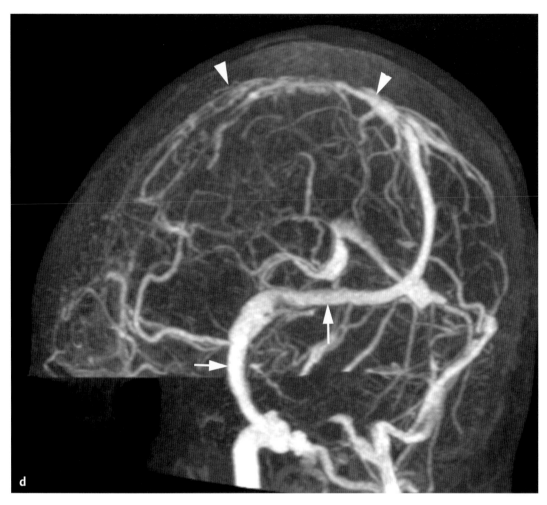

**Fig. 10.29** (*Continued*)  **(d)** Magnetic resonance venogram after treatment shows the sigmoid sinus (*lower arrow*) and transverse sinus (*upper arrow*), as well as a patent superior sagittal sinus (*arrowheads*).

## 10.4.3 Case 3

A young woman of slender build presented with visual loss and headaches. Ophthalmological examination revealed bilateral severe papilledema. Her lumbar opening pressure was noted to be 40 cm of water. Magnetic resonance venography suggested superior sagittal sinus stenosis. After failure of maximal medical therapy, she was considered for venous angioplasty. An over-the-wire balloon was used to dilate the venous stenosis with rapid improvement in vision and headaches and lowering of lumbar opening pressure into the normal range.

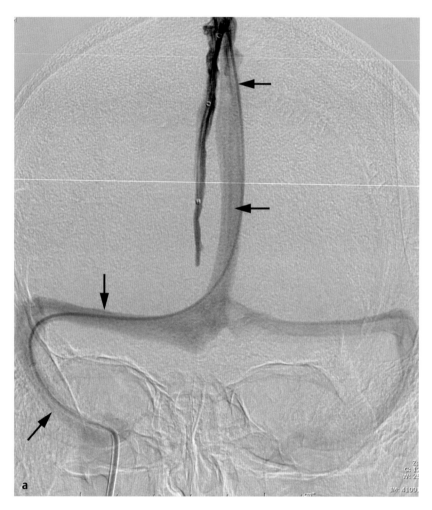

**Fig. 10.30** **(a)** Anteroposterior view of an over-the-wire balloon inserted into the superior sagittal sinus. The wire (*right upper arrow*), superior sagittal sinus (*right lower arrow*), transverse sinus (*left upper arrow*), and sigmoid sinus (*left lower arrow*) are visible.

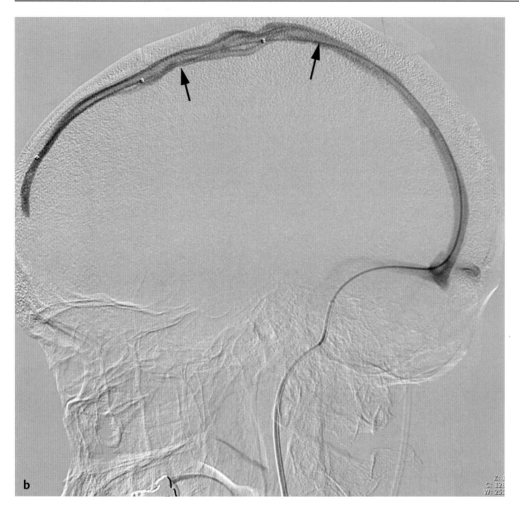

**Fig. 10.30** (*Continued*)   **(b)** Lateral view showing the wire (*right arrow*) and the segment with stenosis (*left arrow*).

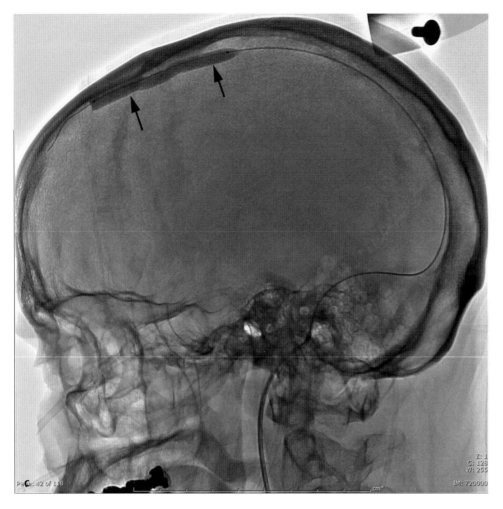

**Fig. 10.30** (*Continued*)    **(c)** Superior sagittal sinus dilated with the balloon (*arrows*).

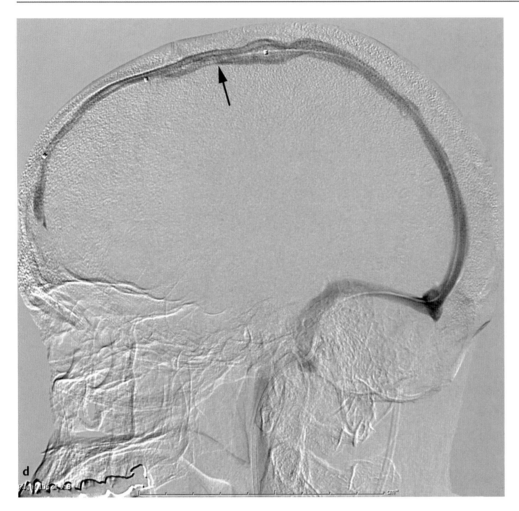

**Fig. 10.30** (*Continued*)   **(d)** Improvement in stenosis (*arrow*) of the superior sagittal sinus.

## Clinical Pearls

### Superior Sagittal Sinus

- The most common pathology affecting the superior sagittal sinus is venous thrombosis. This condition presents a clinical diagnostic challenge because patients present with a many-day history of headaches resulting from increased intracranial pressure because of venous outflow obstruction. The headaches deteriorate with bilateral neurological symptoms, including seizures because of bihemispheric dysfunction. Not infrequently, patients present with a venous hemorrhagic infarct that can be bilateral or unilateral. Prompt diagnosis using magnetic resonance or computed tomographic venography is essential to prevent delays in treatment, which, as for other venous thrombosis in the body, is systemic anticoagulation even in the face of a hemorrhagic infarct. Endovascular intervention is reserved for patients who present in extremis or with impending or ongoing herniation, or who deteriorate further despite adequate systemic anticoagulation.

  The other common pathology affecting any venous structure in the brain, including the superior sagittal sinus, consists of dural arteriovenous fistulas, which are supplied by bilateral external carotid branches, including both scalp and meningeal branches.

  Idiopathic intracranial hypertension is frequently diagnosed in young obese women. However, on occasion, women without morbid obesity can be diagnosed with intracranial hypertension. In these cases, review of sinus anatomy may reveal sinus stenosis that may respond to venous angioplasty and, occasionally, stenting.

### Straight Sinus

- This sinus is severely abnormal, takes atypical routes, and is grossly enlarged in vein of Galen malformations. Thrombosis of the deep venous system, including the vein of Galen and straight sinus, presents with bilateral thalamic edema and venous infarcts with a decreased level of consciousness and bilateral neurological events.

### Transverse Sinus

- The transverse sigmoid junction and superior petrosal sinuses are the most common sites of dural arteriovenous fistulas (AVFs). Dural AVFs are believed to have a predilection for these sinuses because of the likely association with the adjacent petrous bone and mastoid air cells, which can become inflamed as a result of otitis media, causing secondary venous thrombosis with subsequent recanalization resulting in AVF formation. The arterial supply to these fistulas comes primarily from branches of the middle meningeal artery and the transosseous branches of the posterior auricular and occipital arteries. They can be supplied by the meningeal branches of intracranial vessels, such as the artery of Bernasconi-Cassinari arising from the meningohypophyseal trunk of the cavernous carotid artery. During transarterial embolization of the meningeal branches, particularly those that supply the petrous meninges, the geniculate ganglion may be at risk, resulting in facial paresis postembolization.

### Superior Petrosal Sinus

- The superior petrosal sinus can be easily ligated during transtentorial approaches to the upper brainstem in conjunction with presigmoid approaches, such as for anterior petrous and clival masses, which are frequently meningiomas. It is critical to evaluate the drainage of the vein of Labbé draining the temporal lobe when planning these approaches. Typically, the vein of Labbé drains into the transverse sigmoid junction, and in these cases, the petrosal sinus can be easily sacrificed; however, occasionally, the vein of Labbé drains into the distal superior petrosal sinus, and in these cases, ligation of the superior petrosal sinus can result in disastrous venous infarction of the temporal lobe.

  Venous sampling of the superior petrosal sinus may be requested during evaluation of secretory pituitary microadenomas. In these cases, a microcatheter is advanced from the ipsilateral internal jugular vein through the sigmoid sinus and into the ipsilateral petrosal sinus. This test is frequently performed bilaterally to identify asymmetry in location of the pituitary microadenoma.

### Inferior Petrosal Sinus

- The inferior petrosal sinus is the most common route taken to access the cavernous sinus, as may be required during interventional management of carotid cavernous fistulas, both indirect (dural arteriovenous fistulas), as well as direct (trauma or aneurysm). This sinus empties through multiple channels into the anteromedial part of the jugular bulb. Microcatheterization of this sinus allows delivery of coils and liquid embolics safely into the cavernous sinus for transvenous management of carotid cavernous fistulas.

## Sphenoparietal Sinus

- Bridging veins that drain the anterior temporal and inferior posterior frontal lobes frequently drain into this sinus. These veins can be problematic during transsylvian exposure of anterior or posterior circulation aneurysms, obscuring the view or preventing adequate retraction of the frontal and temporal lobes. Although, traditionally, these bridging veins are considered safe for sacrifice, there is concern that there may be cognitive issues and impaired outcomes related to venous injury. Every attempt should be made to preserve these veins, and frequently, meticulous microdissection may prevent the need for their sacrifice

## Cavernous Sinus

- The circular sinus is formed by a circular venous cavity in a dural leaf of the edges of the diaphragma sellae anterior and posterior to the pituitary body forming connections between the two cavernous sinuses. The anterior aspect of the circular sinus is usually larger.

  The cavernous sinus is frequently involved in cavernous carotid fistulas. These can be direct, such as after trauma and laceration of the internal carotid artery or its branches, or after rupture of a cavernous carotid aneurysm. They can also be indirect or dural arteriovenous fistulas fed by branches of both the internal and external carotid artery branches.

  The most common route to the cavernous sinus is through the deep petrosal sinus, although one may access the cavernous through the superior petrosal sinus, or through the pterygoid plexus in the infratemporal fossa, or through the common facial vein, getting access to the superior or inferior ophthalmic vein; and through direct access, either through the inferior orbital fissure or through a cutdown through a superior eyelid incision.

  Engorgement of the cavernous sinus, such as in cases of fistulas or following venous thrombosis, results in chemosis of the ipsilateral or bilateral eyes, as well as cranial neuropathies, primarily affecting the extraocular muscles and causing facial dermatomal pain.

  In cases with severe venous outflow obstruction or hypertension in the orbit, vision may be compromised.

## Vein of Galen

- The prototypical disorder of the vein of Galen is the typically congenital vein of Galen malformation. This is more accurately referred to as a galenic fistula, typically directly fed through fistulous connections from the posterior medial choroidal artery, distal anterior cerebral arteries, as well as splenial and other branches.

# Appendix 1 Diameter of Vessels

| Vessel | Outer diameter of vessel in mm; formalin fixed specimens | |
| --- | --- | --- |
| | Range | Average |
| Basilar artery | 3.2 → 6.5 | 3.96 |
| Superior cerebellar artery, initial segment | 1.0–2.0 | 1.33 |
| Anterior inferior cerebellar artery, initial segment | 0.2–1.5 | 0.88 |
| Posterior inferior cerebellar artery, initial segment | 0.7–3.0 | 1.28 |
| Vertebral artery, intradural segment | (L) 1.65 → 5.25<br>(R) 1.45 → 4.9 | 3.16<br>2.93 |
| Anterior spinal artery | 0.4–1.4 | 0.8 |
| Internal carotid artery<br>    Cranial base<br>    Supraclinoid | <br>4.0–7.0<br>3.0–5.0 | <br>5.3<br>4.0 |
| Ophthalmic artery | 0.7–2.0 | 1.1 |
| Middle cerebral artery<br>    M1<br>    M2<br>    Perforators | <br>2.5–4.9<br>1.0–3.0<br>0.3–1.5 | <br>3.0<br>1.9<br>0.6 |
| Anterior cerebral artery<br>    A1<br>    A2<br>    Heubner's | <br>0.0–3.6<br>1.5–4.0<br>0.5–1.9 | <br>2.9<br>2.7<br>0.94 |
| Anterior choroidal artery, initial segment | 0.5–2.0 | 1.1 |
| Posterior communicating artery<br>    Initial segment<br>    Premammillary artery | <br>0.0–2.5<br>0.4–1.0 | <br>1.5<br>0.7 |
| Posterior cerebral artery<br>    P1<br>    P2 | <br>0.0–3.0<br>2.0–4.0 | <br>2.2<br>2.8 |
| Posterior thalamoperforator | 0.5–1.0 | 0.7 |
| Quadrigeminal artery | 0.3–1.0 | 0.5 |
| Posterior medial choroidal artery | 0.25–1.0 | 0.5 |

# Appendix 2 Laboratory Drawing: Middle Cerebral Artery

Detailed "roadmap" drawing of branches of the right middle cerebral artery. Although some patterns of "roadways" are similar, each middle cerebral artery has a distinct branching pattern. (Louis Bakay Neuroscience Laboratory.)

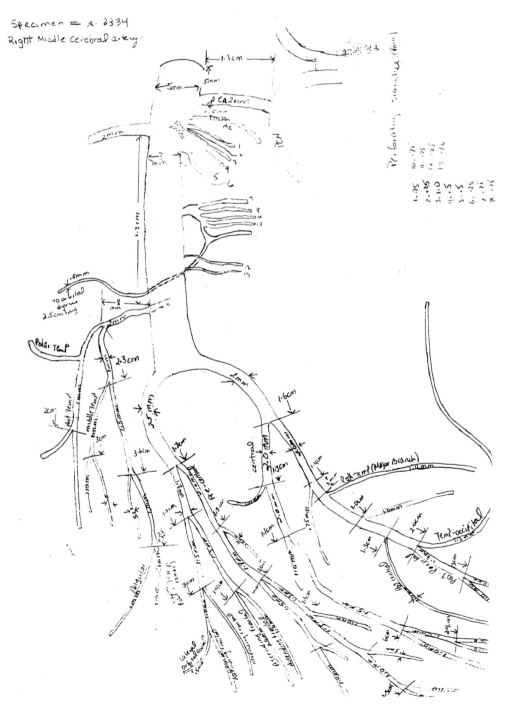

# Index

**285**